Ventricular Assist Devices in Advanced-Stage Heart Failure

Shunei Kyo
Editor

Ventricular Assist Devices in Advanced-Stage Heart Failure

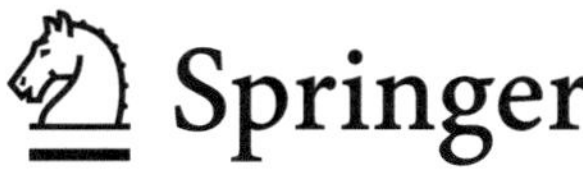 Springer

Editor
Shunei Kyo
Department of Therapeutic Strategy for Heart Failure
The University of Tokyo Hospital
Graduate School of Medicine
The University of Tokyo
Tokyo, Japan

ISBN 978-4-431-56340-2   ISBN 978-4-431-54466-1 (eBook)
DOI 10.1007/978-4-431-54466-1
Springer Tokyo Heidelberg New York Dordrecht London

Springer is part of Springer Science+Business Media (www.springer.com)

Preface

At the end of the nineteenth century, the English surgeon Stephen Paget surmised: "Surgery of the heart has probably reached the limits set by nature; no new methods and no new discovery can overcome the natural difficulties that attend a wound of the heart," expressing how difficult heart surgery was. Doctors as well as average citizens in those days considered the heart to be an untouchable internal organ and believed that a heart operation was impossible. However, Alexis Carrel, who performed a fundamental study of vascular anastomosis at the University of Chicago and established vascular anastomosis technology, transplanted the heart of a young dog to the cervix of an adult dog in 1905 and proved the possibility of recovery of the heartbeat after heart transplantation. Furthermore, Carrel transplanted the heart and lungs of a kitten to the cervix of an adult cat in 1907 and established the fundamental technology of today's heart and heart–lung transplantation. Carrel was awarded the Nobel Prize in physiology or medicine for these achievements in 1912. Additionally, Carrel studied organ preservation and co-authored *The Culture of Organs* with the aviator Charles A. Lindbergh, famous for his solo trans-Atlantic flight of *The Spirit of St. Louis*. Carrel went on to develop the Carrel–Lindbergh Pump, a prototype of today's pump oxygenator, an achievement that was an important step eventually leading to open heart surgery.

By pursuing the possibility of vascular anastomosis and heart transplantation, Carrel introduced the concept that the heart is a repairable and replaceable internal organ, and he was responsible for the concept of mechanical circulatory assist by developing the Carrel–Lindbergh Pump. With these two concepts Carrel established the basis for the fundamental technology that makes today's open heart surgery possible. Open heart surgery is technology that restores valve function and coronary circulation or repairs a congenital defect or structural anomaly of the heart. In open heart surgery, native cardiopulmonary function stops with a surgical operation to the heart. A means (cardiopulmonary bypass) is needed to substitute for systemic circulation normally maintained by the natural heart and lungs.

Clinical introduction of open heart surgery began in the middle of the twentieth century and was carried out through such means as cardiopulmonary bypass, prosthetic valves, and prosthetic grafts, most of which had completely entered the realm of possibility by the end of the century. Artificial heart treatment extends the concepts of surgical repair of the heart by using prosthetic materials and the replacement of the heart by a heart transplant. The artificial heart is in a developmental stage currently, of course, and only ventricular assist devices (VADs) have actually been put into practical use, while the total artificial heart (TAH) is still in the clinical investigation stage. Many functions considered to be "natural" in the natural heart have not yet been completely achieved in the artificial heart. Therefore, long-term survival for more than 10 years for patients supported by VADs has not yet been attained.

In the USA, nearly 2.8 % of the total adult population suffer from heart failure. About 1,100,000 people have been hospitalized every year due to worsening heart failure, and some 280,000 deaths have occurred as a result of heart failure. Approximately 40 billion dollars are spent on medical treatment for heart failure every year in the USA, and it is predicted that heart failure patients and the costs of heart failure treatment will continue to rise. For these reasons, a more effective and efficient treatment strategy for heart failure in medical and surgical treatment must be developed. Although a heart transplant is considered the ultimate therapeutic strategy for heart failure, a heart from a brain-dead donor is not always available at the time it is needed, and their absolute numbers are also extremely limited. The establishment of a medical environment in which end-stage heart failure patients can be assured of treatment when necessary is our mission, and it will be the challenge of the twenty-first century.

Clinical use of the first-generation pulsatile flow implantable left ventricular assist device (LVAD) was introduced in the 1990s and spread during that decade mainly to provide a bridge device to heart transplantation. In 2000, the second-generation continuous flow (CF) implantable LVAD was introduced clinically, and destination therapy was established as a therapeutic alternative to a heart transplant. The main issues to be solved are thrombotic embolism, infection, right heart failure, and a tendency for bleeding. The solution of these challenges is closely connected with improvement in long-term clinical outcome and the improvement of a patient's QOL. With continuous flow implantable LVAD treatment in 2013, we achieved a better prognosis in improving the patient's life for an average of more than 2 years, with the longest survival being more than 8 years. We can predict that the day will soon come when 10-year survival can be achieved with the present devices. Competition is intensifying in the development of the fully implantable LVAD using the percutaneous energy transmission system with which a driveline is not needed. Clinical introduction of the fully implantable LVAD is predicted to be possible by 2020. Improved prognosis, with an expected survival for an average of more than 10 years, will be made possible by clinical introduction of the fully implantable LVAD, and it is predicted that survival for a maximum of 20 years can be achieved by replacing part of the device.

This book commemorates a milestone: With the introduction of destination therapy, the current implantable LVAD has reached the clinical outcome of a 2-year survival rate, almost equivalent to that of heart transplantation for end-stage heart failure. This book is also a "declaration of independence" for the LVAD, marking the starting line from which the implantable LVAD will surpass heart transplantation in prognosis for survival and in QOL in the near future. The time when an artificial heart is considered inferior to a heart transplant soon will come to an end. The day when the status of the artificial heart will have been established as the ultimate therapeutic strategy for end-stage heart failure is at hand.

I had the opportunity to implant a ventricular assist device (the Atsumi–Todai Pump, developed at Tokyo University) in the first Japanese patient in 1980. Thereafter, for more than 30 years, I have been engaged in clinical and research work on the artificial heart. Because performing a heart transplant in Japan was extremely difficult until 1999 due to certain social and cultural factors, a significant delay occurred in the introduction of the implantable LVAD, especially for bridge-to-transplant (BTT) use in Japan. Insurance reimbursement for the implantable CF-LVAD was started in 2011 in Japan. Although it had been delayed for almost 20 years, the artificial heart therapy of Japan with the implantable CF-LVAD ultimately approached the American and European level.

I would like to dedicate this book to the many pioneers in the world who have promoted the development of the artificial heart. Willem J. Kolff, Adrian Kantrowitz, and Michael E. DeBakey in particular are the real parents of the artificial heart. William S. Pierce, Peer M. Portner, and Victor L. Poirier contributed immensely to the development of the ventricular assist device. The Japanese researchers Tetsuzo Akutsu, Yukihiko Nose, and Kazuhiko Atsumi had many great achievements in artificial heart development, and they nurtured numerous researchers who today are playing an active role in Japan and other parts of the world.

Tokyo, Japan   Shunei Kyo

Contents

Abbreviations

ACC	American College of Cardiology
ACGME	Accreditation Council in Graduate Medical Education
ACHF	Advanced chronic heart failure
ADL	Activities of daily living
AHA	American Heart Association
AHF	Advanced Heart Failure
ALVAD	Intra-abdominal left ventricular assist device
AST	Aspartate aminotransferase
AST/SGOT	Aspartate Aminotransferase/serum glutamic oxaloacetic transaminase
BCBS	Blue Cross Blue Shield
BiVAD	Biventricular assist device
BNP	Brain natriuretic peptide
BP	Blood pressure
BTT	Bridge to Transplantation
BUN	Blood urea nitrogen
CAV	Coronary allograft vasculopathy
CDC	Centers for Disease Control and Prevention
CEA	Cost effective analysis
CFD	Computational fluid dynamic
CF-LVADs	Continuous flow left ventricular assist devices
cGMP	Cyclic guanine monophosphate
CHF	Congestive Heart Failure
CMS	Center for Medicare and Medicaid Services
CO	Cardiac output
CPB	Cardiopulmonary bypass
CPR	CardioPulmonary Resuscitation
CRT	Cardiac resynchronization therapy
CTICU	Cardiothoracic Intensive Care Unit
CVP	Central venous pressure
DT	Destination Therapy
DTRS	Destination therapy risk score

ECMO	Extracorporeal membrane oxygenation
EF	Ejection fraction
ESP	Evidence-based Synthesis Program
FDA	Food and Drug Administration
FFP	Fresh frozen plasma
FILVAS	Fully Implantable Ventricular Assist System
GI	Gastrointestinal
HF	Heart failure
HMWM	Higher Molecular Weight Multimers
HRPCI	High-risk percutaneous coronary interventions
IABP	Intra-aortic balloon pumping
ICD	Implantable cardioverter-defibrillator
ICER	Institute for Continuing Education and Research
iNO	Inhaled nitric oxide
INR	International normalized ratio
INTERMACS	Interagency Registry for Mechanically Assisted Circulatory Support
ISHLT	International Society of Heart and Lung Transplantation
IVS	Interventricular septum
JCAHO	Joint Commission on Accreditation of Healthcare Organizations
J-MACS	Japanese registry for Mechanically Assisted Circulatory Support
KCCQ	Kansas City Cardiomyopathy Questionnaire
LDL	Low-density lipoprotein
LOE	Level of evidence
LV	Left ventricle
LVAD	Left Ventricular Assist Device
LVEF	Left Ventricular Ejection Fraction
MCS	Mechanical Circulatory Support
MEDPAR	CMS Medicare Provider Analysis and Review
METS	Metabolic Equivalent Task Score
MLHF	Minnesota Living with Heart Failure
MLWHF	Minnesota Living with Heart Failure
MRI	Magnetic resonance imaging
mTOR	Mammalian target of rapamycin
6MWD	6-Minute walk distance
6-MWT	6-Minute walk test
NHLBI	National Heart, Lung, and Blood Institute
NT	N-terminal
NYHA	New York Heart Association
OHC	Open heart centers
PAP	Pulmonary artery pressure
PCWP	Pulmonary capillary wedge pressure
PHP	Percutaneous heart pump
PSI	Percutaneous site infections
PVR	Pulmonary vascular resistance
QALY	Quality adjusted life year

QUERI	Quality Enhancement Research Initiative's
RAP	Right atrial pressure
RCA	Pulmonary vascular resistance
REMATCH	Randomized Evaluation of Mechanical Assistance for the Treatment of Congestive Heart Failure
RV	Right ventricle
RVAD	Right ventricular assist device
RVEF	Ejection fraction of the right ventricle
RVF	Right ventricular failure
RVFAC	RV Fractional area change
RVOT	RV outflow tract
RVSP	RV systolic pressure
RVSWI	RV stroke work index
SIRS	Systemic inflammatory response syndrome
TAPSE	Tricuspid valve (TV) annular plane systolic excursion
TC	Transplant center
TEE	Transesophageal echocardiography
TET	Transcutaneous energy transmission
TR	Tricuspid regurgitation
TV	Tricuspid valve
UNOS	United Network for Organ Sharing
VAD	Ventricular Assist Device
VO2	Oxygen consumption
vWF	von Willebrand Factor

Chapter 1
Opportunities and Challenges for LVAD Therapy Now and in the Future

Walter P. Dembitsky and Robert M. Adamson

Abstract Left ventricular assist devices (LVADs) are increasingly being used to support patients suffering from advanced heart failure. Efficacy has been proven in prospective controlled trials. Observations from registries and clinical experiences all suggest improving mortality, morbidity, and costs. Global expansion of the technology serves as tacit endorsement of these notions. The large gap between actual and projected potential use can be partially explained by improvements in medical therapy for heart failure and heart transplantation as well as the biological limitations of the implanted machines and their relationship to the retained native heart . Improvements in the near future will focus improving clinical management strategies and the introduction of full implantable systems. Ultimately pumps which have a more intimate relationship both to the retained heart and host will be necessary to improve results. This will include the introduction of pulsatility and the reduction of shear stress and the use of more bio-friendly materials.

Keywords Left ventricular assist device (LVAD) • LVAD biocompatibility • LVAD clinical problems • LVAD native heart interrelationship • LVAD utilization

1.1 Introduction

1.1.1 The Current Landscape

The demographics of the world's population is changing. During the 1950s, the preponderance of populations were composed of younger people with few over the age of 65. By the year 2050, in Europe, Japan, and China, there are projected to be

W.P. Dembitsky (✉) • R.M. Adamson
Sharp Memorial Hospital, San Diego, CA, USA
e-mail: dembitsky@aol.com

S. Kyo (ed.), *Ventricular Assist Devices in Advanced-Stage Heart Failure*,
DOI 10.1007/978-4-431-54466-1_1, © Springer Japan 2014

                                          W.P. Dembitsky and R.M. Adamson

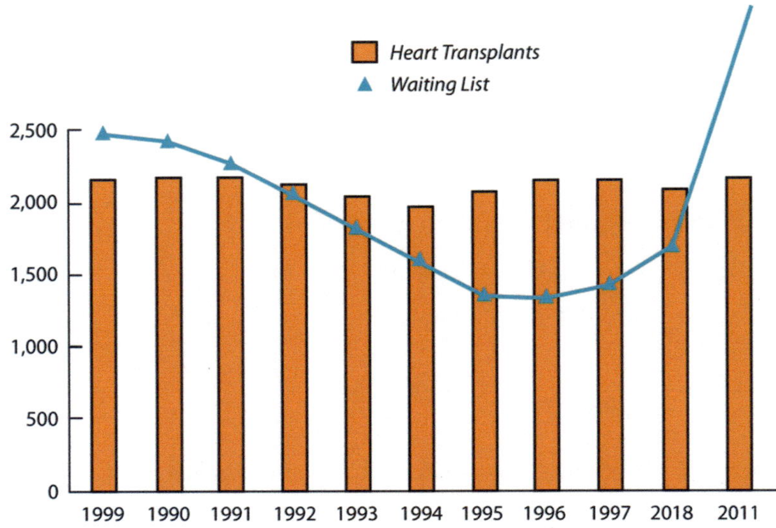

Fig. 1.1 Number of transplants and size of active waiting list

more people over the age of 65 than under the age of 20 [1]. During the erstwhile phases of industrialization, most deaths were caused by communicable diseases and accidents. Currently, in industrialized countries, most deaths are caused by degenerative diseases such as cancer and cardiovascular disease, including heart failure. The prevalence of heart failure by age and gender rises from about 1 % between age 40 and 50 in the USA to almost 12 % in patients over the age of 80. In patients in the age range of 60–80, approximately 9 % of men and 5 % of women will have heart failure, giving a total prevalence of approximately 5.7 million in the year 2008. Furthermore, from 1970 to 2008, the new cases per year have increased from 250,000 to approximately 670,000 [2].

In association, there has been a fourfold increase in hospital discharges in age over 65 years from the years 1970 to 2008 [3]. This increase has been associated with a hierarchy of treatment strategies. In stage D heart failure with refractory symptoms requiring special interventions, the suggested interventions are chronic inotropic infusion, left ventricular assist device implantation, heart transplantation, or finally, terminal care such as the hospice system in the USA. Heart transplantation has been resource limited and had its peak application in the USA in the 1990s. Since then, slightly over 2,000 heart transplants are performed each year. Other countries in the Asian Pacific region are beginning to explore heart transplantation as a resource to treat terminal heart failure but as yet, the experience is limited. The total number of transplants performed worldwide in 2010 was slightly less than 4,000. The size of the waiting list in the USA has actually begun to rise and, in 2011, far exceeded that of the number of patients transplanted as seen in Fig. 1.1 [4].

This rise is attributable to the increasing number of waiting patients bridged with mechanical circulatory support devices. In the USA, approximately one-third of patients transplanted are actively supported by left ventricular assist devices. In

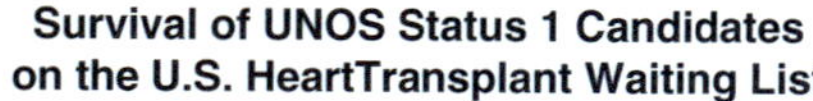

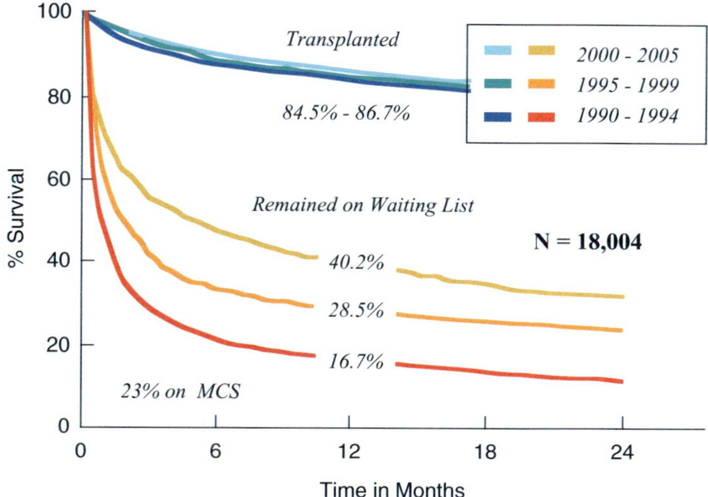

Fig. 1.2 Survival of UNOS Status I candidates on the US Heart transplant waiting list

some communities in the USA, 100 % of patients transplanted are supported by ventricular assist devices.

In an attempt to expand the donor pool, the mean age of donors has increased. In the USA, the mean age of donors has risen from 25 years in 1988 to 27 years in 2010. In Europe, the mean age of donors is now approximately 41 years of age. Concomitant with the attempt to expand the donor pool and increasingly supporting patients with ventricular assist devices, the survival of UNOS Status I candidates on the US Heart transplant waiting list has gradually improved. The survival at 12 months of UNOS Status I candidates from 1990 to 1994 was 16 %, from 1995 to 1999 survival has risen to 28.5 %, and during the early part of the current era from 2000 to 2005 it has risen to 40.2 % (Fig. 1.2). Of that surviving group, 23 % were on mechanical circulatory support systems. Of those transplanted, survival at 1 year was 84–87 %.

The survival of UNOS Status II candidates has also improved (Fig. 1.3). From 1990 to 1994, the 12-month survival rate was 65 %, from 1995 to 1999 it was 72 %, and from 2000 to 2005 it was 80 %. Ninety percent to 93% of those patients transplanted survived at 1 year [5].

The improvement in survival of medically treated Status II candidates now rivals the 1-year survival of the transplanted patients. Thus, the primary indication for transplantation of Status II patients is to improve their quality of life. The survival of heart transplant recipients has also slowly improved by era. The half-life in the decade from 1982 to 1992 was eight and one-half years, from 1993 to 2002 it was 10.9 years, and from 2000 to 2006 the survival was slightly improved; although half-life has not yet been reached, survival at seven years is approximately 64 %. The survival at 2 years has improved from approximately 70 to 81 % over the time period described (Fig. 1.4).

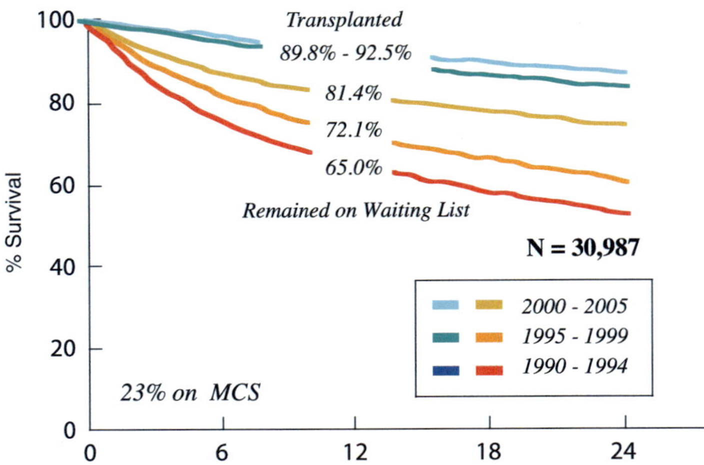

Fig. 1.3 Survival of UNOS Status II candidates on the US Heart transplant waiting list

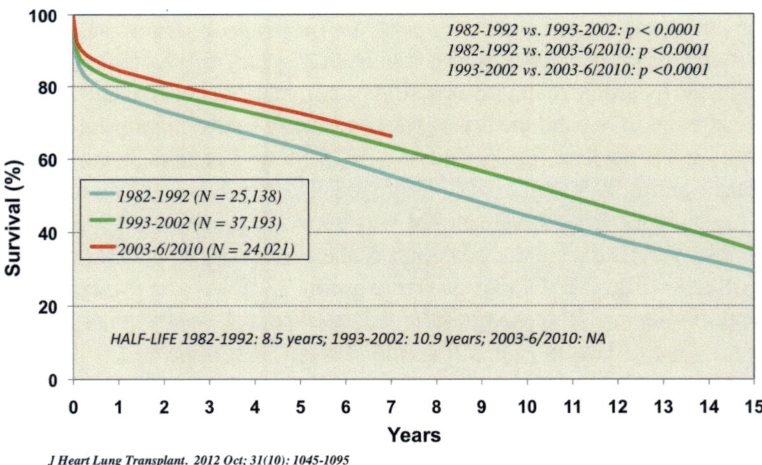

Fig. 1.4 Kaplan-Meier survival by era, adult heart transplants

The pivotal Rematch Study compared an optimally managed medical group before the era of resynchronization therapy to the survival of a group implanted with a pulsatile HeartMate I LVAD. The prospective control trial showed a dramatic improvement in survival for the LVAD arm, from 8 % to approximately 25 % at 2 years [6]. Subsequent trials comparing the HeartMate II continuous flow pump to the pulsatile HeartMate I predecessor demonstrated improved survival of 68 % at 2 years [7]. Individual centers now report 2-year survival of 80 % with ventricular assist device-supported patients [8]. This rivals transplantation at a 2-year time period.

No randomized trials currently exist comparing transplant patients to medical therapy or to long-term LVAD therapy, so all conclusions in this domain are based on comparative observations. Nonetheless, the 2-year efficacy for using LVADs to treat terminal heart failure has been proven. And now, initial explorations are being made trying to assess whether LVADs for destination therapy are on track to compete with heart transplantation. As recently reported by Kirklin [9], certain important subsets of patients, comprising 20 % of patients receiving continuous flow destination therapy, now enjoy a 2-year survival competitive with heart transplantation. The worldwide clinical experience of left ventricular assist device has increased dramatically and in 2013 over 14,000 patients have been implanted with a variety of devices. Currently, most patients have been implanted with the HeartMate II continuous flow pump. The increased global distribution of ventricular assist device implantations is tacit endorsement of the technology's efficacy. In 2005, the USA, Canada, and five countries in Europe were implanting devices. The devices have now been implanted on every major continent, including South America, India, Eurasia, Asian Pacific, and Australia.

The estimated potential number of patients with ventricular assist device implants under the age of 70 in the USA is about 30 per 100,000. It has been further estimated that about 7 cases per 100,000 in the USA are added annually [10]. Comparing 2010–2011, in the 20 largest metro systems in the USA, the number of patients implanted is far below these projected numbers [11].

In summary, the heart failure landscape in 2013 shows a continued universal organ shortage and improved medical outcomes. There have been slight improvements in transplant outcomes and new rotary pumps provide improved 1- and 2-year survival. Their acceptance is increasing but has so far been less than projected.

1.2 Current Opportunities for Improvement

1.2.1 The Problem

There is a disparity between estimated need for LVADs and their actual application. The gap is likely due to the perceptions of quality of life, especially as influenced by real and perceived mortality, morbidity, and costs.

We analyzed the costs of transplantation in our own center and compared them to LVAD insertion. It was found that the cost of LVAD insertion declined by 40 % over a 5-year study period, while the cost of heart transplantation rose 12 %. Half of the LVAD implantation cost was the cost of the device. Interestingly, the causes of death for the LVAD population were largely a progression of other diseases. In contrast, the deaths in the transplant population were mostly attributable to immune-related maladies, often induced, such as neoplasm, infection, and graft rejection.

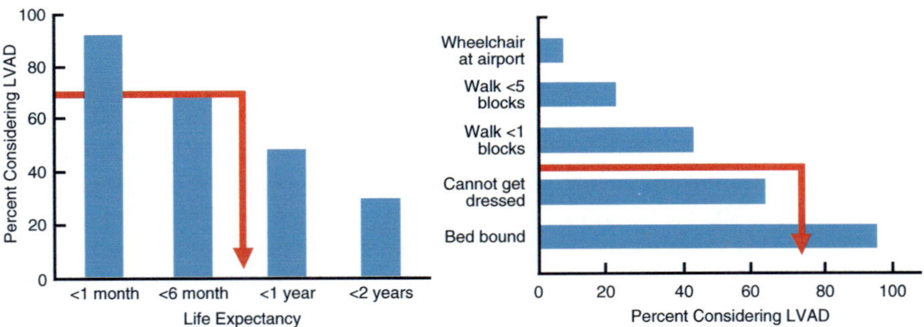

Fig. 1.5 Thresholds of physical activity and life expectancy for patients considering destination ventricular assist devices

The importance of quality of life has been addressed by many and in the article by Stewart [12] about 60 % of patients with heart failure, quality of life was as important as survival. About 25 % felt that the quality of life was more important than survival and a few felt survival was more important than quality. In general, younger patients do prefer to live longer and older patients prefer to live better. Stewart determined what thresholds for physical activity and life expectancy currently prompt patients to consider an LVAD destination device. About 70 % of patients who felt that their life expectancy was about 8 months would consider themselves to be eligible for a left ventricular assist device. When asked "would you consider an assist device to be more active?," 70 % of patients would consider an assist device if they could not dress themselves (Fig. 1.5).

Over the reported 2-year time course of LVAD implant studies, functional capacity and quality of life do improve. The six-minute walk distance, New York Heart Association Functional Classification, metabolic equivalent task score, Minnesota Living with Heart Failure Score, Kansas City Cardiomyopathy Score, and neurocognitive function all improve significantly following implantation of a HeartMate II and HeartWare assist devices. NYHA functional class was determined by an independent clinician at the time points shown [13]. Improvements were statistically significant in both trials ($p < 0.001$) [14–19]. Despite these proven advantages, real problems continue to influence the quality of life for recipients. If an implantable device had no associated mortality or morbidity, acceptance thresholds would certainly lower.

Hospital readmissions do have an adverse effect on quality of life. Using INTERMACS database, Kirklin assessed the readmission rate for over 2,000 LVAD recipients [20]. About half the patients had no readmissions, 22 % had one readmission and many patients had multiple admissions (Fig. 1.6).

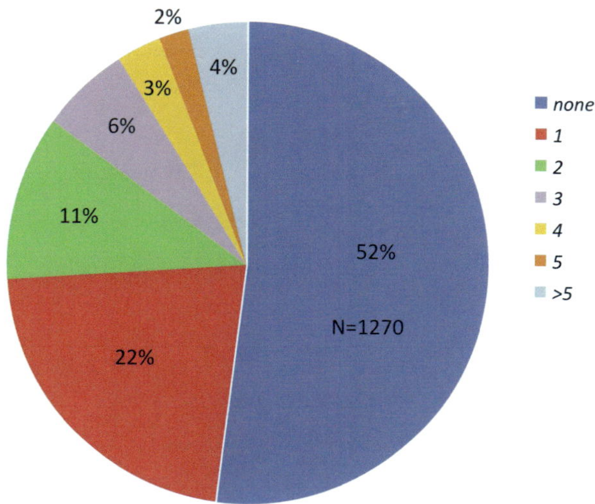

Fig. 1.6 LVAD readmissions

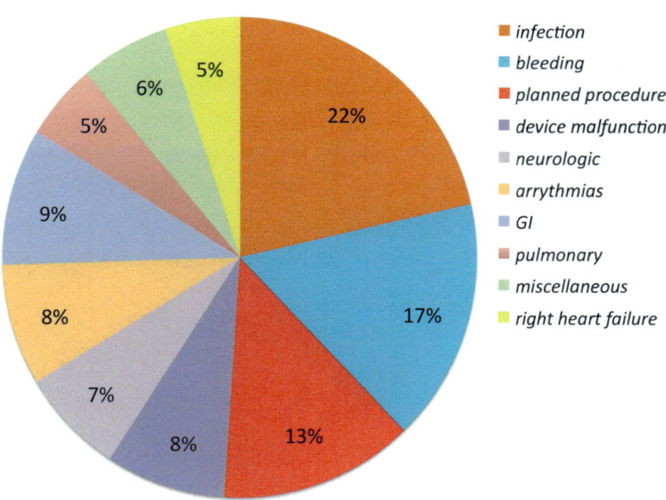

Fig. 1.7 LVAD readmission causes

The most common cause was infection. The second most common cause was bleeding, followed by application of planned procedures such as pacemakers, ablations, and finally, a myriad of other problems including neurological, gastrointestinal, and pulmonary. Five percent of readmissions were due to right heart failure (Fig. 1.7).

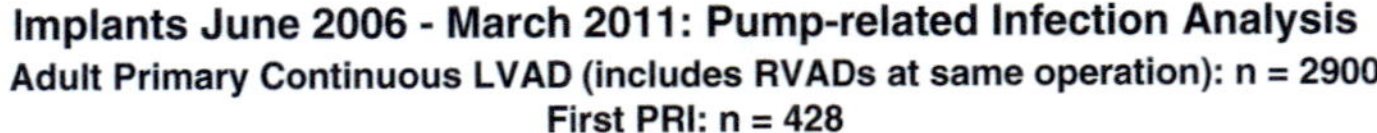

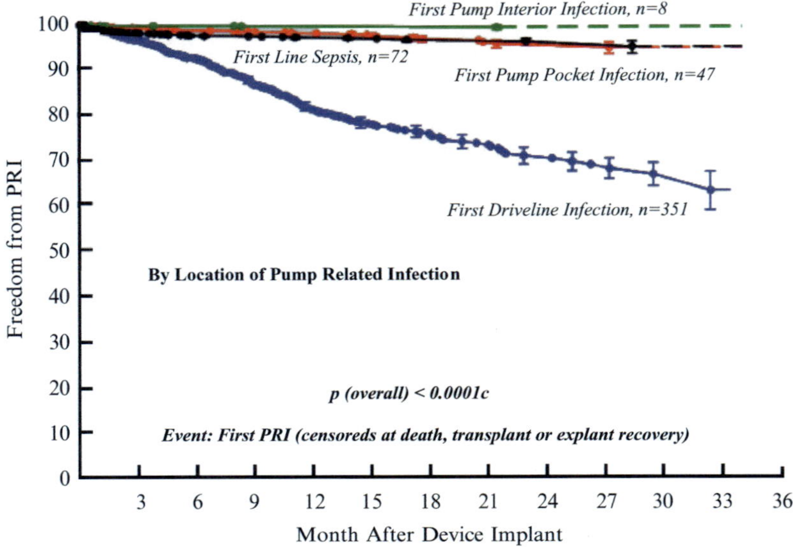

Fig. 1.8 Implants June 2006–March 2011: pump-related infection analysis

The driveline infection curve shows a slope (Kirklin) that is continuous, reflecting a constant incidence of this problem (Fig. 1.8).

Overall, the occurrence of more serious internal pump infections, driveline sepsis, and pocket infections remain small. All are related to the liability of an implanted artificial surface.

1.3 Infection

1.3.1 The Solution

Standard definitions for infectious problems are being formulated in an attempt to ascertain the best way to prevent and treat them. Our own efforts have been published and have served as a reasonable guide for some [21]. The biomaterial interface is especially vulnerable as it passes through the skin where it is exposed to trauma and hostile bacteria. Future application of more bio-friendly surface technologies may help circumnavigate this problem. In the near future, fully

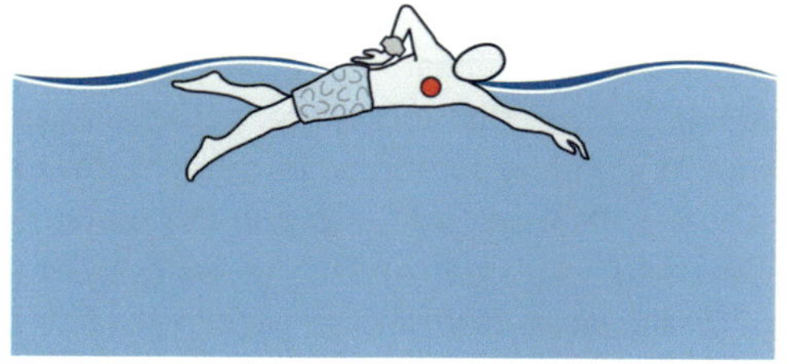

Fig. 1.9 Three hours untethered support—no percutaneous drive line

implantable HeartMate II left ventricular assist device pumps will be available for use. A major advantage of fully implantable device systems is replacing the percutaneous drive line by using a transcutaneous energy transmission system. In order to achieve reasonable energy transmission efficiency these systems initially required close proximity of the inducting and receiving coils on and in the patient's body. With the introduction of newer energy transmission systems, such as WiTricity, the devices are now able to be located more remotely in the body without severe loss of transmission efficiency. With the initial systems, superimposition of coils was important to achieve 80 % energy transmission efficiency. If the patients were to gain weight and increase the distance from the coils, the efficiency could be reduced to 50 %. Experience with these transcutaneous systems was reported during the early LionHeart implant fully implantable left ventricular assist device and the AbioCor fully implantable total artificial heart device. The current goal for a Thoratec is to have 3 h of untethered support time which will attenuate to 2 h after 2,000 cycles, representing approximately 2 years of recharges.

Using these systems will improve patient's quality of life by allowing additional freedoms such as bathing and swimming. More importantly, in fully implantable systems, infection rates are expected to be reduced (Fig. 1.9).

1.4 Thrombosis, Thromboembolism, Hemolysis, and Bleeding

Pump thrombosis, hemolysis, bleeding, and thromboembolism are all attributable to the inherent design characteristics of the continuous flow pumps. All are influenced by the interplay of recipient patient characteristics, implantation techniques, and management styles. There is no doubt that all of these hematologic liabilities are induced by the addition of an LVAD. Rotary continuous flow devices disturb the homeostatic state of the circulating blood by creating high shear stress levels and areas of non-laminar, even static flow conditions in the retained native heart.

Initial recommendations for anticoagulation and anti-aggregation strategies were made capriciously. Platelets were known to be activated by levels of shear stress exceeding 100 dynes. The high shear stress created by rotary pumps seemed to warrant the administration of antiplatelet drugs. Aspirin was recommended. Now, aspirin has been implicated in gastrointestinal bleeding in patients receiving coronary stents [22]. Furthermore, the well-documented loss of the high molecular weight von Willebrand multimer in rotary LVAD recipients creates platelet dysfunction. These facts bring into question the wisdom of using anti-aggregation medications for HMII.

Since stasis is known to occur with continuous flow conditions, anticoagulation with Coumadin seemed appropriate. This notion was reinforced by the high pump thrombosis rate of the early model of the MicroMed DeBakey-Noon pump [23].

Now, the routine use of Coumadin is being scrutinized. Certain subsets of patients seem to be more prone to bleeding than to thrombosis. In these patients, increased anticoagulation using Coumadin may be a liability. In our own experience of patients with bleeding abnormalities requiring cessation of anticoagulation, over 20 patients have fared well with no increased thrombotic complications for over 1 year.

The incidence of hemorrhagic and embolic strokes has been higher in females than in males. Younger patients seem to be more susceptible to thromboembolism. During the latter half of the continued access protocol for the HeartMate II, destination therapy trial experience anticoagulation levels were lowered. The incidence of hemorrhagic stroke was diminished, but the less morbid embolic stroke rate was not increased [24]. The origin of systemic embolization is often from the aortic outflow tract including the supra- and subvalvular regions and probably from embolic material generated within the pump.

The incidence of first stroke gradually increases with time. In the INTERMACS database at 36 months, 81 % of patients were free of stroke, and 92 % were free of pump thrombosis (Fig. 1.10).

Pump thrombosis (Fig. 1.11) can be difficult to diagnose and the treatment and prevention has not been well defined. It currently felt that thrombosis can be the result of an ingested clot generated in the retained heart or by clot formed locally within the pump. Preventive strategies must address the coagulability of the individual host as well as the prothrombotic flow conditions that the pumps induce in themselves as well as in the host. The latter can be adversely influenced by odd apical cannula positions which restrict flow.

Changes in current demands can be indicators of impending thrombosis if the thrombus creates drag on the rotor. Flow-restricting thrombus external to the rotor may not produce current changes. The use of flow sensors on rotary device conduits would be most helpful for diagnosing and predicting pump thrombosis. The additional information would hopefully serve as a guide for the more effective use of preemptive therapeutic lytic therapies.

Flow aberrations created by constricted areas of flow including clot formation in or around rotors can dramatically increase the rate of hemolysis in patients supported by continuous flow pumps. The hematologic cost of producing continuous flow is high. Flow architecture and recirculation, and high shear stress effects on blood elements, all function over time to create abnormalities. These abnormalities

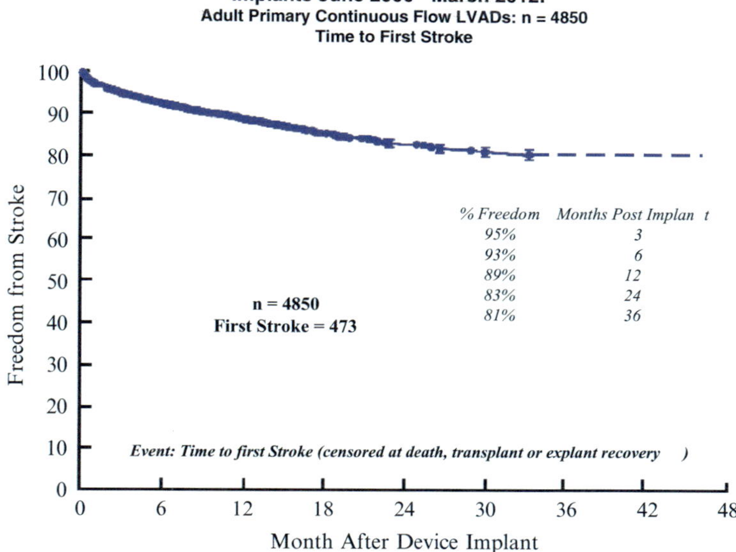

Fig. 1.10 Implants June 2006–March 2012: adult primary continuous flow LVADs

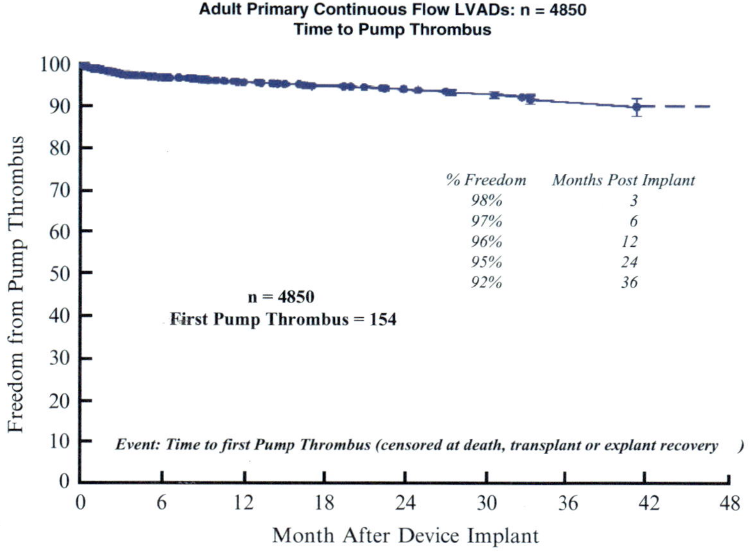

Fig. 1.11 Implants June 2006–March 2012: adult primary continuous flow LVADs; time to pump thrombus

are tolerated to different degrees by different hosts. Since all left ventricular assist devices are recirculating devices, the flow history becomes more important over time [25]. The exposure to high shear stress history is dramatically increased in

LVAD patients who have aortic insufficiency. This increases the instantaneous shear stress but also, by virtue of the central recirculation of blood, the flow history. Continuous flow pumps can be made to generate higher pressures, but they do so at the cost of increased shear stress. This may tax the hematologic shear stress tolerance of the individual host. This is dictated by the resilience of the formed elements (i.e., the presence of spherocytosis induced or acquired), hepatic and renal reserves coupled with the ability of the bone marrow to respond and compensate for reduced red blood cell survival times. When shear stress is over 2,000 dynes, red blood cells are destroyed. This hemolysis may be related to thrombosis since products of red cell lysis promote thrombin generation. Red cell survival studies in patients with bileaflet valves show that red cell survival is diminished from 120 to 100 days. In vivo red cell survival has not been measured to date with left ventricular assist devices but is surely low. Platelet activation occurs at greater than 50 dynes/cm^2, with lysis over 100 dynes/cm^2 and fragmentation over 250 dynes/cm^2. Normal shear stress in biological systems ranges from 10 dynes/cm^2 in the venous system to 70 dynes/cm^2 in the systemic arterial circulation [26].

1.5 Improving Management Styles

The length of stay following device implantation, 30-day mortality, 1 year survival, gastrointestinal bleeding, driveline infection rates, stroke rates, use of inotropes, and hemolysis varied greatly across practices in the USA. An analysis using the INTERMACS database for 17 centers, each with over 50 patients for a total of 1,234 patients, revealed that one may excel in one or more areas but not in others (Table 1.1). This has prompted the use of a Best Practices Initiative to try to standardize therapies with the expectation that results will improve.

The challenge during the next decade for LVAD patients will be that new assessments of efficacy will be applied. A new time metric will be necessary. During the era when left ventricular assist device survival was unusual, 2 years was thought to be more than enough time to validate device applications. Now, quality of life and survival beyond 5 years is becoming increasingly important. Currently, almost 100 patients have survived over the 5-year period and some for as long as 10 years on multiple devices with good qualities of life. The new extended time metric will create new challenges. Infection, thrombosis, thromboembolism, bleeding, device failure, and native heart deterioration all increase over time and will contribute to accumulating costs and degradation of quality of life. To meet this challenge, it will be important to maintain and improve quality, not only of technology, but of management styles.

Unless management styles change, the infrastructure needed to support implanted LVAD patients may increase beyond manageable levels in the not too distant future (Fig. 1.12). In 2011, 3,150 patients were implanted and there were 4,500 patients treated as outpatients. In 2015, if 10,000 patients are implanted, the infrastructure requirements to support a potential 20,000 outpatients will be enormous.

Table 1.1 Thoratec best practices initiative; implants April 2008–September 2011: follow-up as of December 2013

Center	% Age >60	% DT	Average Intermacs profile	Avg. LVAD duration	LOS	30-day mortality (%)	1-year survival(%)	GI bleed (%)	DL infection (%)	Stroke (%)	RVF (RVAD) or inotropes (%)	Hemolysis (%)
Median	39	20	2.5	324	20	4	81	10	13	6	6	3
Min	27	6	1.9	206	13	0	76	4	5	0	0	0
	58	56	4.3	451	30	9	91	19	24	16	53	14

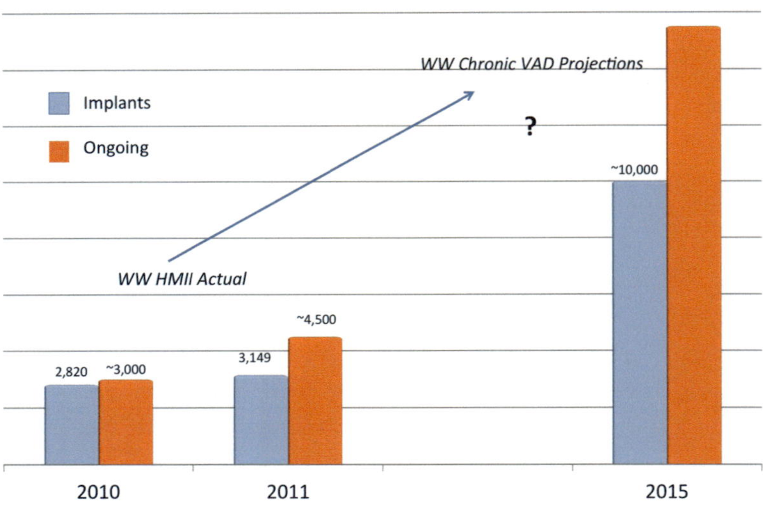

Fig. 1.12 Increasing infrastructure requirements

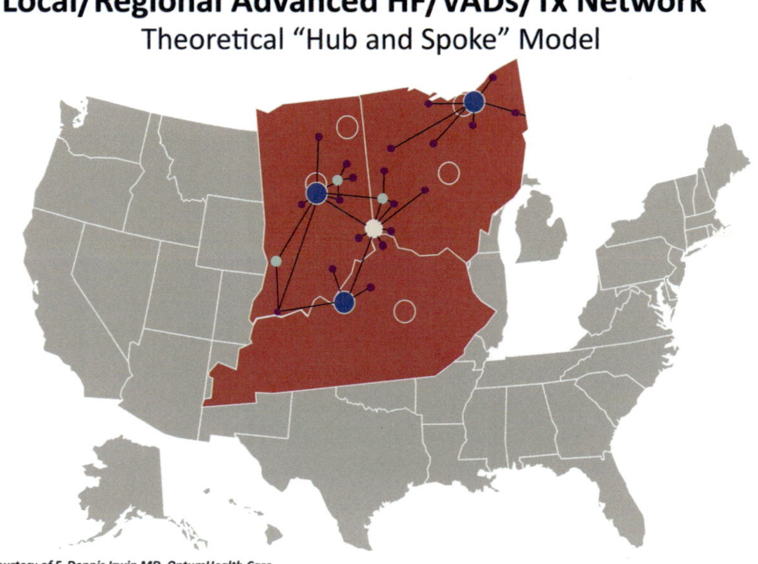

Fig. 1.13 Local/regional advanced HF/VADs/Tx network

One promising management style is the shared hub and spoke model where more sophisticated implanting centers are able to manage patients in cooperation with referring centers (Fig. 1.13).

1.6   Designing the Perfect Pump

Even with the above variables optimized, the inherent liabilities of the current technology remain. Perfect pumps to support a biological system do exist. Design queues are evident when considering the results of the natural experiment with circulatory support in biological systems which began in multicellular animals seven hundred and 50 million years ago. Disparate branches of the phylogenetic tree with complex circulatory designs have evolved to the same position, separated pulmonary and systemic circulations powered by pulsatile sequential volume displacement pumps. This example of convergent evolution is an endorsement of a good design. At the apex of the invertebrate phylogenic chain are the cephalopods which have a divided circulation with pulsatile flow. Squid have a single left ventricle and two right ventricles, each with pulsatile flow. Birds and mammals are the most advanced vertebrates. They also have separate pulsatile circulations. These divided circulations have evolved to create higher sustained systemic pressures and flows with the ability to change pressures and keep volumes constant. The pumps used in natural systems are volume displacement pumps which propel fluid by inducing thrust in which a decreasing chamber size expels fluid through an aperture, and the position of the chamber is moved along with the fluid that it contains. Industrial pump manuals offer a functional description of a form of volume displacement pumps which have a diaphragm. They continue to flow independent of pressure. There are no seals, close fittings, sliding, or rotating parts. There is no heat buildup in confined areas. There is minimal degradation of viscosity of shear sensitive material. There is a low suction relative to discharge pressures and they require valves to create unidirectional flow. All of these latter pump characteristics are optimized in advanced biological circulatory systems and impedance matching seems to be the rule (Fig. 1.14).

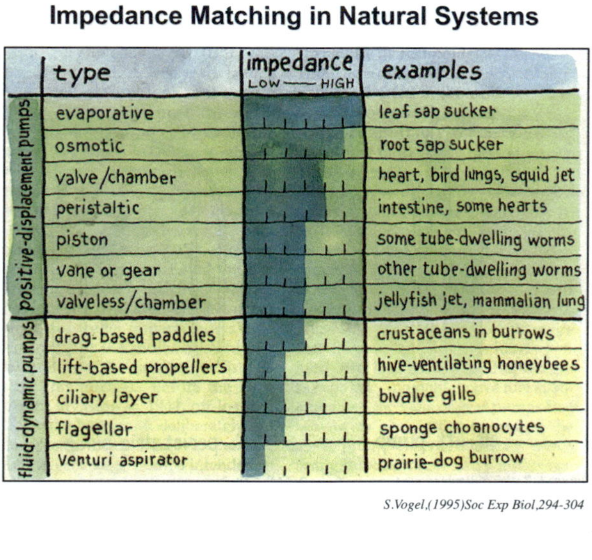

Impedance Matching in Natural Systems

	type	impedance LOW —— HIGH	examples
positive-displacement pumps	evaporative		leaf sap sucker
	osmotic		root sap sucker
	valve/chamber		heart, bird lungs, squid jet
	peristaltic		intestine, some hearts
	piston		some tube-dwelling worms
	vane or gear		other tube-dwelling worms
	valveless/chamber		jellyfish jet, mammalian lung
fluid-dynamic pumps	drag-based paddles		crustaceans in burrows
	lift-based propellers		hive-ventilating honeybees
	ciliary layer		bivalve gills
	flagellar		sponge choanocytes
	Venturi aspirator		prairie-dog burrow

S.Vogel,(1995)Soc Exp Biol,294-304

Fig. 1.14 Impedance matching in natural systems [27]

Alternatively, continuous flow pumps can be generally characterized as fluid dynamic. When used for circulatory support, they propel blood by spinning it or by radial force. The two pump types, fluid dynamic and volume displacement, have profoundly different characteristics. In general, fluid dynamic rotary pumps are volume pumps and volume displacement pumps are pressure pumps. Across the wide experience of natural pumping systems, impedance matching is generally found where fluid dynamic pumps are used for volume and volume displacement pumps are used to create pressure [27].

Fluid dynamic pumps have distinct advantages especially when viewed from an engineering perspective. There are fewer moving parts. No compliance chamber is necessary. They are more durable, more efficient, and less expensive. They are easier to implant because of the smaller size. They have less surface area and they are more quiet. Biologically they have the disadvantages of having a high inlet pressure, being pressure limited, and they create high shear stress and areas of stasis. Finally, they are associated with attenuated or no pulsatility.

It is no surprise that the adverse consequence of high shear stress and attenuated pulsatility is now being witnessed in ongoing clinical applications of continuous flow circulatory support pumps to biological circulatory systems so well adapted to volume displacement pumps. A problem for the future will be describing exactly what is meant by pulsatility. The rate and duration of pulsatility, its relationship to compliance and resistance, and its relative importance in biological systems have not been well defined. Similarly, the hematologic effects of high shear stress and the limits of individual host tolerance must be explored.

1.7 Repair the Native Heart and Then Add an LVAD

Even if an implantable left ventricular assist device can be designed by engineers, which is truly forgettable from a patient's perspective, the retained native heart remains as a potential source of problems. It is capable of imposing severe maladies which will affect both the quantity and the quality of life of the LVAD recipient. For that reason, our own practice has been to correct the native heart and then to add an LVAD. Most of our recipients have had at least one additional procedure and some have had many (Fig. 1.15). Valve repairs are the most common associated procedure (Fig. 1.16).

Average cardiopulmonary bypass time for simple pump insertion is about 20 min. Total average time for patients receiving additional procedures is about 80 min. This is time well spent, especially as chronic LVAD support becomes the norm.

1.8 Right Heart Dysfunction

The right heart with increased demands of higher cardiac output and potential changes in the intraventricular septal geometry can produce increasing degrees of tricuspid insufficiency which might already be present in patients with severe heart

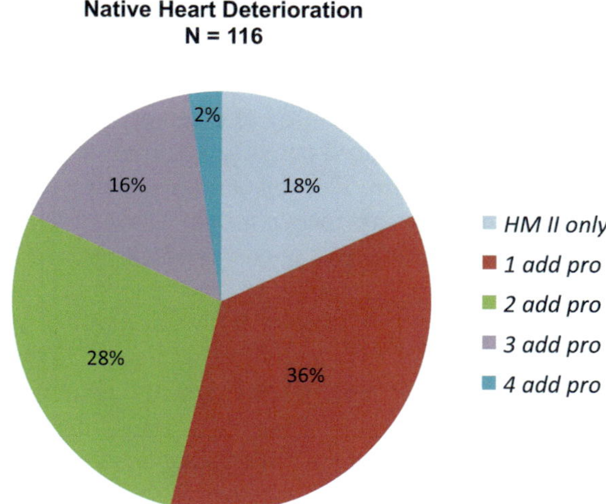

Fig. 1.15 Sharp additional procedures to prevent native heart deterioration

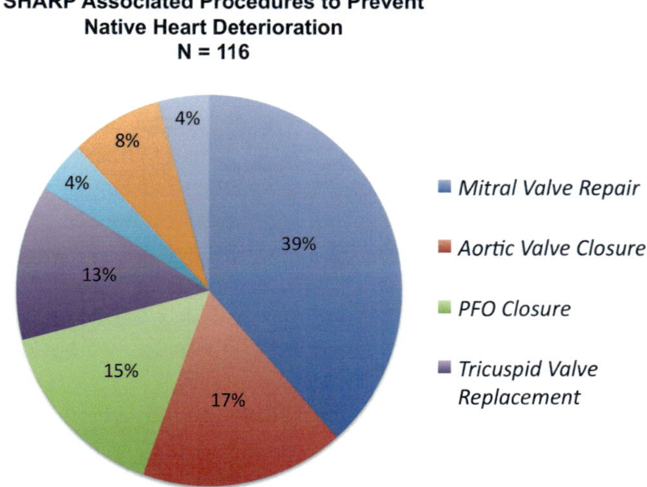

Fig. 1.16 Sharp associated procedures to prevent native heart deterioration

failure at the time of the implantation. This is especially the case in patients with previously placed trans-tricuspid valvular leads which can cause scarring and destruction of the valvular mechanism. Often, this can be corrected initially with valvuloplasty techniques but may require tricuspid valve replacement. The right ventricle, like the left, can become a source of ventricular arrhythmias late in the course following LVAD implantation.

In a minority of patients, right-sided pumping may be necessary. In our own early experience with pulsatile pumps, the high end of exercise capacity was limited by the ability of the left ventricular complex to perform but not the ability of the right ventricle to pump [28]. This may also be the case with continuous flow pumps. In some patients with high PVR, the ability of a compromised RV pump may not provide sufficient flow to the left-sided pumping complex or may do so at the cost of a high systemic venous pressure. This Fontan-like condition might be improved with biventricular pumping. The presence of an additional pump will create liabilities. The use of implantable biventricular continuous flow systems has been tried on a limited basis [29, 30].

On the left side of the heart, ventricular arrhythmias may also be a problem late in the course of the disease. They are usually well tolerated and do not significantly effect long-term survival. Implantable defibrillators and ablative therapies can be helpful [31, 32].

The arrhythmias can have epicardial origins and postoperatively they can be extremely difficult to ablate. During implantation, on the left side, preemptive ablations connecting scars to apical cannula sites, especially in patients with ischemic cardiomyopathy, might ameliorate the late tendency to develop arrhythmias, although this is unproven.

1.9   Left Heart Dysfunction

The native heart on the left side can present hemodynamic abnormalities and flow geometry disturbances which can predispose the patient to hemolysis, heart failure, and thromboembolism. The most vexing area in patients chronically supported with left ventricular assist devices is the left ventricular outflow tract. Using rotary pumps, the continuous flow nature of the blood returned into the aortic root predisposes the root to retention of static recirculating flow areas which have been shown to produce both thrombus and thromboembolism into the systemic circulation, including the brain and the coronary arteries. Furthermore, we have demonstrated that in patients with continuous flow devices, especially those with severely reduced left ventricular function, flow is directed from the mitral valve to the apex of the ventricle. This unusual intraventricular flow pattern creates a static recirculation gyre in the outflow tract which we have seen to be thrombogenic and has a high stasis index [33]. Thromboembolism is linked to intraventricular flow stasis in a patients supported with left ventricle assist devices.

Finally, the aortic valve which has evolved over many millions of years spends approximately half of its time in systole and is now obliged to spend all of its time in diastole. The liabilities of this new biological role are as yet undefined for certainty. However, aortic valve insufficiency does increase with time of left ventricular assist device support, and the incidence of aortic insufficiency in an LVAD population, described by Ragagopal [34], is greater than in the clinically treated heart failure population. As seen in Table 1.2 [35–39], the incidence varies from 25 % to as high as 75 % at a 12-month interval.

Table 1.2 Incidence of aortic insufficiency during LVAD support

Author	Incidence %	Population	Time interval (months)	Risk factors
Soleimani	32	66 HMII HeartWare	12	DT status Age >1 year support
Toda	38	47	12	Preop MR Less AoV opening
Pak	25	130 HM I–II	12	CF pump Preop Ao root dil Less AoV opening
Hatano	70	37	2–18	CF devices Lower EF Less AoV opening
Cowger	51	13 CF and PF	12–18	AoV opening, Ao Diameter, lower lv Volumes

The risk factors which seem to be related to the occurrence of aortic valvular regurgitation are those associated with abnormal tissue integrity such as mitral regurgitation, dilation of the aortic root, and advancing age. Reduced opening of the aortic valve during LVAD support has also been implicated [40]; however, patients who acquire aortic insufficiency may open the valve less, making conclusions regarding etiology less certain. In our experience of 98 HeartMate II patients known to be free of significant aortic insufficiency at the time of implantation, 12 % of the patients at 27 months (range 12–51 months) were reoperated upon for congestive heart failure due to aortic insufficiency. This high failure rate must be addressed to assure the best long-term outcomes for patients. The etiology of the insufficiency remains undefined. The high transmural gradient may produce abnormal nutritional flow to the valve. Furthermore, the lack of shear stress across the ventricular aspect of the valve with the increased strain on the valve all may be involved with protein signaling which predisposes the valve to fibrosis. In our analysis [41, 42], we were able to demonstrate a fibrotic reaction of the ventricular aspect of aortic valves in patients supported long-term with left ventricular assist devices. The aortic aspect of the valve remained normal. The mechanical strain on the aortic valve does influence fibroblast extracellular matrix and potential for stenosis in native aortic valves and these factors may, indeed, be especially implicated in patients reported with LVAD [43].

The implications of these changes and the liability they impose will demand closer attention to the aortic root in the future. Aortic insufficiency increases the recirculation time and, hence, the exposure history for red cells. This is manifested by an increasing hemolysis rate. Furthermore, depending on the native ventricular function and competency of the mitral valve, the aortic insufficiency produces higher end-diastolic pressures which can ultimately produce right heart failure. This intolerable induced abnormality can be addressed at the time of surgery by closing the aortic valve using the Adamson technique [44].

Percutaneous correction of aortic insufficiency in LVAD recipients has been variably successful. Sapien and CoreValve transfemoral valves as well as Amplatzer occluder devices have all been attempted with some reported success [45, 46].

We have had catastrophic failure with an Amplatzer device and feel that, generally, device retention in the aortic root can be problematic if aortic sclerosis is not present.

It is also known that pulsatile flow pumps create aortic insufficiency, although it appears that the incidence of root thrombosis was less with pulsatile pumps than continuous flow pumps.

We currently advocate repairing the mitral valve in patients implanted with LVADs if the regurgitation is greater than 2+ and especially if the annulus is dilated. This is simply accomplished with a vent in the ventricular apical cannulation site with a non-ischemic beating heart. Mitral insufficiency during periods of LVAD support produces a potential liability because the contracting ventricle reduces the pulsatility index by ejecting as some of the flow is ejected back through an incompetent mitral valve instead of through the apex of the heart. Finally, device explantation in a patient who has mitral insufficiency requiring repair is more complex. Therefore, in the future, our strategy of correcting native heart abnormalities and then adding a ventricular assist device will serve patients best.

The left atrium can be a source of embolization. In patients with atrial fibrillation, the left atrial appendage should be amputated.

1.10   Optimizing Flow Patterns

To date, bulk flow has been the primary way of measuring the contribution of LVADs to the host. However, it is well known that normal bulk flow with abnormal flow geometry in conditions such as atrial fibrillation, aortic aneurysm, and dilated cardiomyopathy can be associated with the disturbances of local flow architecture which cause stasis and recirculation which are thrombogenic. Therefore, even in natural systems which malfunction, anticoagulation is required. In any implanted intravascular machine, the requirement for anticoagulation or aggregation therapy is a manifestation of a design defect. In the future, in order to obtain singularity with biological design, almost surely pulsatility and reduced shear stress will be important. Achieving this goal is likely to encompass growing information technologies which allow synchronization of continuous flow pumps to the native system and hopefully the development of durable pulsatile systems that do not increase shear stress which may not be well tolerated in compromised hosts.

References

1. United Nations, Department of Economic and Social Affairs. Population division, population estimates and projections section. UN DESA; 2013.
2. Circulation. 2012;125(1):e2–e220 and 2010 National Heart Lung and Blood Institute Fact Book.
3. Jessup M, Brozena S. The American heart association and the American college of cardiology general guidelines for treatment of systolic heart failure as presented by Jessop in 2003. N Engl J Med. 2003;348:2007–18.

4. OPTN/SRTR. Annual Report, Tables 1.7, 11.1a 2009.
5. Leitz M. Improved survival of patients with end-stage heart failure listed for heart transplantation: analysis of organ procurement and transplantation network/U.S. United Network of Organ Sharing Data, 1990 to 2005. J Am Coll Cardiol. 2007;50(13):1282–90.
6. Rose R et al. Long-term mechanical left ventricular assist for end-stage heart failure. N Engl J Med. 2001;345:1435–43.
7. Slaughter MS et al. Advanced heart failure treated with continuous-flow left ventricular assist device. N Engl J Med. 2009;361:2241–51.
8. Kirklin JK, Naftel DC, Pagani FD, Kormos RL, Stevenson L, Miller M, Young JB. Long-term mechanic circulatory support (destination therapy): on track to compete with heart transplantation? J Thorac Cardiovasc Surg. 2012;144(3):584–603; discussion 597–8. doi:10.1016/j.jtcvs.2012.05.044.
9. Kirklin JK et al. J Thorac Cardiovasc Surg. 2012;144:584–603.
10. Jevenandum V. Thoratec users meeting; 2007.
11. Oconell J. Thoratec users meeting; 2012.
12. Stewart GS, Brooks K, Pratibhu PP, et al. Thresholds of physical activity and life expectancy for patients considering destination ventricular assist devices. J Heart Lung Transplant. 2009;28(9):863–9.
13. Rogers JG, Aaronson KD, Boyle AJ, Russell SD, Milano CA, Pagani FD, Edwards BS, Park S, John R, Conte JV, Farrar DJ, Slaughter MS; HeartMate II Investigators. Continuous flow left ventricular assist device improves functional capacity and quality of life of advanced heart failure patients. J Am Coll Cardiol. 2010;55(17):1826–34. doi: 10.1016/j.jacc.2009.12.052.
14. Rogers JG, Aaronson KD, Boyle AJ, et al. Continuous flow left ventricular assist device improves functional capacity and quality of life of advanced heart failure patients. J Am Coll Cardiol. 2010;55(17):1826–34.
15. Abraham WT, Fisher WG, Smith AL, et al. Cardiac resynchronization in chronic heart failure. N Engl J Med. 2002;346:1845–53.
16. Rector TS, Cohn JN. Assessment of patient outcome with the Minnesota living with heart failure questionnaire: reliability and validity during a randomized, double-blind, placebo-controlled trial of pimobendan. Am Heart J. 1992;124:1017–25.
17. Rector TS, Kubo SH, Cohn JN. Validity of the minnesota living with heart failure questionnaire as a measure of therapeutic response to enalapril or placebo. Am J Cardiol. 1993;71:1106–7.
18. Spertus J, Peterson E, Conard MW, et al. Monitoring clinical changes in patients with heart failure: a comparison of methods. Am Heart J. 2005;150:707–15.
19. Majani G, Giardini A, Opasich C, et al. Effect of valsartan on quality of life when added to usual therapy for heart failure: results from the Valsartan Heart Failure Trial. J Card Fail. 2005;11:253–9.
20. Kirklin JK et al. Long-term mechanical circulatory support (destination therapy): on track to compete with heart transplantation? J Thorac Cardiovasc Surg. 2012;144:584–603.
21. Chinn R, Dembitsky W, Eaton L, Chillcott S, Stahovich M, Rasmussen B, Pagani F. Multicenter experience: prevention and management of left ventricular assist device infections. ASAIO J. 2005;51(4):461–70. *Source*: Sharp Memorial Hospital, San Diego, CA USA. Park S, et al. Circ Heart Fail. 2012.
22. Hsiao FY, Tsai YW, Huang WF, Wen YW, Chen PF, Chang PY, et al. A comparison of aspirin and clopidogrel with or without proton pump inhibitors for the secondary prevention of cardiovascular events in patients at high risk for gastrointestinal bleeding. Clin Ther. 2009;31(9):2038–47. doi:10.1016/j.clinthera.2009.09.005.
23. Jahanyar J, Noon GP, Koerner MM, Youker KA, Malaisrie SC, Ngo UQ, et al. Recurrent device thrombi during mechanical circulatory support with an axial-flow pump is a treatable condition and does not preclude successful long-term support. J Heart Lung Transplant. 2007;26(2):200–3. *Source*: Michael E. DeBakey Department of Surgery, Baylor College of Medicine, Houston, Texas 77030, USA. jahanyar@bcm.tmc.edu.

24. Park S et al. Outcomes in advanced heart failure patients with left ventricular assist devices for destination therapy. Circ Heart Fail. 2012;5:241–8.
25. Girder G, Bluestein D. Biological effects of dynamic shear stress in cardiovascular pathologies and devices. Expert Rev Med Devices. 2008;5(2):167–81.
26. Girder G, Bluestein D. Biological effects of dynamic shear stress in cardiovascular pathologies and devices. Expert Rev Med Devices. 2008;5(2):167–81.
27. Vogel S. Impendence matching in natural systems. Soc Exp Biol. 1995;294–304.
28. Jaski BE, Lingle RJ, Reardon LC, Dembitsky WP. Left ventricular assist device as a bridge to patient and myocardial recovery. Prog Cardiovasc Dis. 2000;43(1):5–18.
29. Cleveland JC Jr et al. Survival after biventricular assist device implantation: an analysis of the Interagency Registry for Mechanically Assisted Circulatory Support database. J Heart Lung Transplant. 2011;30(8):862–9. doi:10.1016/j.healun.2011.04.004. Epub 2011 May 31.
30. Cleveland JC Jr et al. Survival after biventricular assist device implantation: an analysis of the Interagency Registry for Mechanically Assisted Circulatory Support database. J Heart Lung Transplant. 2011;30(8):862–9. doi:10.1016/j.healun.2011.04.004. Epub 2011 May 31.
31. Boyle A. Arrhythmias in patients with ventricular assist devices. Curr Opin Cardiol. 2012;27(1):13–8. doi:10.1097/HCO.0b013e32834d84fd.
32. Boyle A. Curr Opin Cardiol. 2012;27(1):13–8. doi:10.1097/HCO.0b013e32834d84fd.
33. May-Newman K, Wong K, Adamson R, Hoagland P, Dembitsky W. Thromboembolism is linked to intraventricular flow stasis in a patient supported with a left ventricle assist device. ASAIO J. 2013;59(4):452–5.
34. Rajagopal K et al. Impact of left ventricular assist device implantation upon native aortic valve regurgitation. J Heart Lung Transplant. 2012;31:S261–2.
35. Toda K, Fujita T, Domae K, Shimahara Y, Kobayashi J, Nakatani T. Late aortic insufficiency related to poor prognosis during left ventricular assist device support. Ann Thorac Surg. 2011;92(3):929–34. doi:10.1016/j.
36. Cowger J, Pagani FD, Haft JW, Romano MA, Aaronson KD, Kolias TJ. The development of aortic insufficiency in left ventricular assist device-supported patients. Circ Heart Fail. 2010;3(6):668–74. doi:10.1161/CIRCHEARTFAILURE.109.917765.
37. Pak SW, Uriel N, Takayama H, Cappleman S, Song R, Colombo PC, et al. Prevalence of de novo aortic insufficiency during long-term support with left ventricular assist devices. J Heart Lung Transplant. 2010;29(10):1172–6.
38. Naka Y, Jorde UP. Prevalence of de novo aortic insufficiency during long-term support with left ventricular assist devices. J Heart Lung Transplant. 2010;29(10):1172–6.
39. Soleimani B, Haouzi A, Manoskey A, Stephenson ER, El-Banayosy A, Pae WE. Development of aortic insufficiency in patients supported with continuous flow left ventricular assist devices. ASAIO J. 2012;58(4):326–9.
40. Hatano M, Kinugawa K, Shiga T, Kato N, Endo M, Hisagi M, et al. Less frequent opening of the aortic valve and a continuous flow pump are risk factors for postoperative onset of aortic insufficiency in patients with a left ventricular assist device. Circ J. 2011;75(5):1147–55.
41. May-Newman K. Biomechanics of the aortic valve in the continuous flow VAD-assisted heart. Am Soc Artif Intern Organs J. 2010;56:301–8.
42. May-Newman K et al. Geometry and fusion of aortic heart valves from pulsatile flow ventricular assist device patients. J Heart Valve Dis. 2011;20:149–58.
43. Lehmann S, et al. Mechanical strain and the aortic valve: influence on fibroblasts, extracellular matrix, and potential adamson. Ann Thorac Surg. 2009;88:1476–83; J Heart Lung Transplant 2011;30(5):576–82
44. Adamson et al. J Heart Lung Transplant. 2011;30(5):576–82.
45. D'Ancona G, Pasic M, Buz S, Drews T, Dreysse S, Hetzer R, et al. TAVI for pure aortic insufficiency in a patient with a left ventricular assist device. Ann Thorac Sug. 2012;93(4):e89–91.
46. Grohmann J, Blanke P, Benk C, Schlensak C. Trans-catheter closure of the native aortic valve with an Amplatzer Occluder to treat progressive aortic regurgitation after implantation of an left-ventricular assist device. Eur J Cardiothorac Surg. 2011;39(6):e181–3.

Chapter 2
The State of Ventricular Assist Device Therapy Today

Erskine A. James and John B. O'Connell

Abstract Despite advances in most cardiovascular care, heart failure remains a predominant problem in industrialized nations, with significant mortality, morbidity, and associated costs. The development of left ventricular assist devices, first as a bridge to transplant and then as destination therapy, has significantly improved survival and quality of life of patients with end-stage heart failure. Initial durable ventricular assist devices were large pulsatile devices, but later models have become much smaller, more effective, and more durable as continuous-flow pumps, both axial and centrifugal flow. While these devices have some risk of complications and current models require anticoagulation, patients' overall quality of life and survival have been significantly affected in a positive way. As patient survival has improved, the growth of implantation and care of LVAD patients has created a paradigm of "hub and spoke" model for transplant centers and non-transplant open heart centers to improve access and care to patient for left ventricular assist devices.

Keywords Axial flow • Centrifugal flow • HeartMate II • Mechanical circulatory support • Shared care

2.1 Introduction

Despite significant improvements in the treatment of most cardiovascular diseases, heart failure (HF) remains a significant problem in medical care in the industrialized nations with prevalence rising. In the USA, HF afflicts more than six million (4 % of the adult population) and is the most common cause of hospitalization after normal

E.A. James (✉) • J.B. O'Connell
The Heart Failure Center, The Georgia Heart Center, The Medical Center of Central Georgia, Mercer University School of Medicine, 777 Hemlock Street, MSC #53, Macon, GA 31201, USA
e-mail: james.erskine@mccg.org

S. Kyo (ed.), *Ventricular Assist Devices in Advanced-Stage Heart Failure*,
DOI 10.1007/978-4-431-54466-1_2, © Springer Japan 2014

childbirth. Hospital discharges have risen and now exceed one million for primary HF diagnosis and three million for primary or secondary diagnosis in the USA per year. The 30-day readmission rate is approximately 25 % with more than half being admitted before seeing a physician in follow-up after discharge. The estimated cost exceeds $39 billion. As a result, 34 cents of every dollar spent by Medicare (mostly over age 65 years) goes toward HF care. The 5-year mortality for heart failure is approximately 50 % with 30-day mortality of approximately 12 % among Medicare patients [1].

In Japan, there are more than two million suffering from HF which accounts for more than 170,000 annual deaths. Readmission rates are 35 % at 1 year and the annual mortality for HF with reduced ejection fraction (EF) in NYHA Class III and IV is 35 % [2]. This problem is of comparable epidemiologic significance in both the East and the West.

2.2 Advanced Heart Failure Therapies

The treatment of chronic HF is evidence-based [3], yet it is expected that when presenting with NYHA Class III and IV, less than half will respond to neurohormonal and device-based therapy [4]. Yet, in Japan less than half of the HF population is optimized on medical therapy [2]. Those not responsive (persistently symptomatic and unable to perform activities of daily living (ADLs) despite maximally tolerated medical therapy who have objective evidence of left ventricular (LV) dysfunction and objectively reduced function capacity, as defined by a six-minute walk test distance less than 300 m or peak VO2 less than 12–14 mL/kg/min), fall into the category of "advanced heart failure" (AHF) [5] (Table 2.1).

This population represents those who have HF with preserved EF with tenuous fluid balance, cardiac resynchronization therapy (CRT) nonresponders, those who tolerate suboptimal doses of neurohormonal inhibition due to hypotension or cardiorenal syndrome, those requiring oral diuretic dosages greater than 1.5 mg/kg equivalent of furosemide, intravenous diuretics, or addition of thiazides to loop diuretics, and those requiring intravenous inotropes at any point, recurrent hospitalizations for HF, recurrent appropriate implantable cardioverter–defibrillator (ICD) discharges, persistent symptoms with ADLs, and multiple complex comorbidities. Therapeutic options for these patients include further optimization of medical therapy or addition of CRT (which may or may not be effective), high-risk conventional cardiac surgery, cardiac transplantation, bridge to transplant (BTT) or destination therapy (DT) ventricular assist device(VAD), or palliative care.

2.3 The Evolution of Mechanical Circulatory Support

While cardiac transplantation remains the treatment of choice for patients with AHF, application of this procedure has not made a difference epidemiologically in the management of this population. In the USA, there have been no more than 2,000–2,400 transplants (~2.0/100,000 population) performed each year for the last

Table 2.1 Definition of advanced heart failure (AHF) [5]

1. Severe symptoms of HF with dyspnea and/or fatigue at rest or with minimal exertion (NYHA functional class III or IV)
2. Episodes of fluid retention (pulmonary and/or systemic congestion, peripheral edema) and/or of reduced cardiac output at rest (peripheral hypoperfusion)
3. Objective evidence of severe cardiac dysfunction, shown by at least one of the following:
(a) A low LVEF (<30 %)
(b) A severe abnormality of cardiac function on Doppler echocardiography with a pseudo-normal or restrictive mitral inflow pattern
(c) High LV filling pressures (mean PCWP>16 mmHg and/or mean RAP>12 mmHg by pulmonary artery catheterization)
(d) High BNP or NT-proBNP plasma levels, in the absence of noncardiac causes
4. Severe impairment of functional capacity shown by one of the following:
(a) Inability to exercise
(b) 6-MWT distance <300 m or less in females and/or patients aged ≥75 years
(c) Peak VO2 < 12–14 mL/kg/min
5. History of ≥1 HF hospitalization in the past 6 months
6. Presence of all the previous features despite "attempts to optimize" therapy including diuretics, inhibitors of the renin–angiotensin–aldosterone system, and beta-blockers, unless these are poorly tolerated or contraindicated, and CRT, when indicated

ACHF advanced chronic heart failure, *NYHA* New York Heart Association, *LV* left ventricular, *EF* ejection fraction, *PCWP* pulmonary capillary wedge pressure, *RAP* right atrial pressure, *BNP* brain natriuretic peptide, *NT* N-terminal, *6-MWT* 6-minute walk test, *VO2* oxygen consumption, *CRT* cardiac resynchronization therapy [5]

23 years (Fig. 2.1) due to a severe shortage of acceptable donor organs [6]. However, given the 3.1 million in the USA with HF and low EF, which represents 50 % of overall HF population, 8–10 % of which have AHF and conservatively excluding 75 % for aggressive therapy due to lack of family support, noncompliance, substance abuse, or neurocognitive deficits, the need for advanced heart failure options approaches 30/100,000 population or 93,000, a figure never to be achieved by heart transplantation which currently provides donors to ~1/100,000. In Japan, with an estimated population of HF with low EF slightly over one million, the estimated need using similar assumptions is approximately 18/100,000 population or 23,000! Yet, heart transplantation is performed at a far lower per capita rate and the wait for a suitable donor organ typically exceeds 800 days. Keeping potential recipients alive until a suitable donor is identified is a challenge to say the least worldwide.

Although the first successful VAD was implanted following post-cardiotomy pump failure as a bridge to recovery, the stimulus to develop the field was the inappropriate death rate on the transplant list because of the severity of illness and the long wait until a donor was identified. The advent of left mechanical circulatory support (MCS) with VADs has been a crucial component in improving the lives of those waiting for a transplant and hence the first indication was BTT. Since most will wait from months to several years, MCS must be considered long-term implantation and those not considered transplant candidates may benefit from DT. Initial pulsatile devices, while improving survival and cardiac output, were large and bulky devices with poor durability and a propensity for thrombosis, and as such, had limited application worldwide.

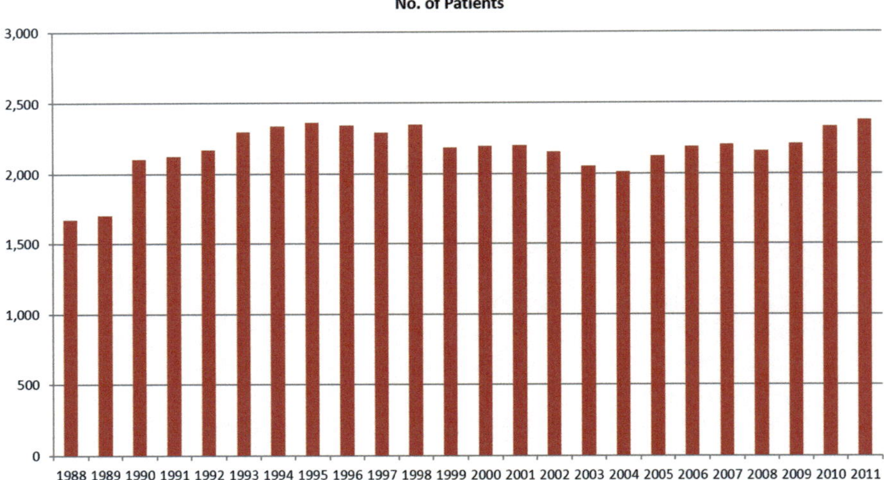

Fig. 2.1 Heart transplants in the USA [6]

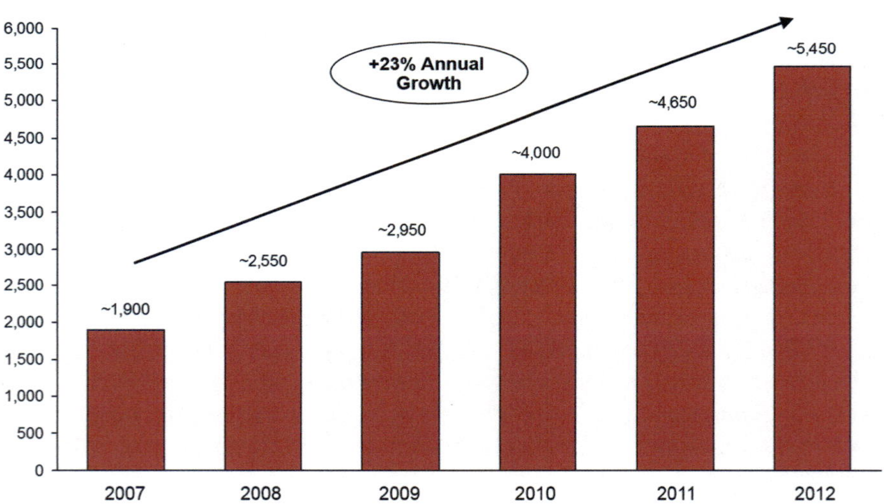

Fig. 2.2 Worldwide HeartMate II LVAD implantation [7]

However, in the US REMATCH study, there was a significant and dramatic difference in survival at 24 months between those receiving the HeartMate XVE and those randomized to medical therapy to the point that despite the poor durability of the pump, it was approved by the US FDA for DT (see below). Newer continuous-flow devices have been proven superior to medical care in clinical outcomes and quality of life. As such, following approval of the HeartMate II initially for BTT and now for DT, VADs are being used more and more frequently worldwide [7] (Fig. 2.2).

2.4 LVAD in Practice

2.4.1 Pulsatile Pumps

The first durable LVAD devices were pulsatile pumps such as Novacor (World Heart) and HeartMate XVE (Thoratec). These devices were electrical pumps similar to paracorporeal devices such as the Toyobo Heart, with the advantage of the durable VAD having the pump itself internalized, so patients could be discharged home from the hospital. The HeartMate XVE was approved for both BTT and DT in 2001 and 2003 in the USA, respectively. The HeartMate XVE was a large device comprised of the internal pump and the external controller and batteries. The internal pump, made from titanium predominantly, had a blood chamber, motor chamber, driveline, and inflow and outflow conduits. The pump weighed 1,150 g, and each conduit had a porcine valve within the Dacron graft. The XVE had a maximum stroke volume of 83 mL and could operate up to 120 beats per minute, which could generate flows of up to 10 L/min. The blood and motor chambers were separated by a unique membrane of textured polyurethane, which prevented thrombus formation. The size of this device required a patient to have a body surface area of at least 1.5 m^2.

2.4.1.1 Rematch Trial

The randomized evaluation of mechanical assistance for the treatment of congestive heart failure (REMATCH) trial was the pivotal trial in the initial use of VADs, which compared medical therapy to mechanical support in AHF. Patients in this trial were eligible if they were patients with AHF, as defined as a peak oxygen consumption of no more than 14 mL/kg of body weight per minute or continuous need for intravenous inotropic therapy, and ineligible to receive heart transplantation, and were randomized 1:1 XVE or continued medical therapy. The findings of this trial showed that the medical therapy arm had a survival of 25 % at 1 year and an 8 % survival at 2 years. This mortality rate was higher than the rates of breast, lung, and colon cancer and acquired immunodeficiency syndrome [8]. Survival was significantly improved in patients who received a HeartMate XVE with a 1-year survival of 52 % and 2 years of 23 %, with a median survival of 408 days. The most common causes of death in the device group were sepsis at 41 % and device failure of 17 %. These findings led to the HeartMate XVE approval for DT in 2003.

2.4.2 Continuous-Flow Axial Flow Pumps

The next evolution in durable VADs is a significant change from the older model of pulsatile pumps. These newer pumps are continuous-flow pumps which have the advantages of being significantly smaller as well as greater mechanical reliability

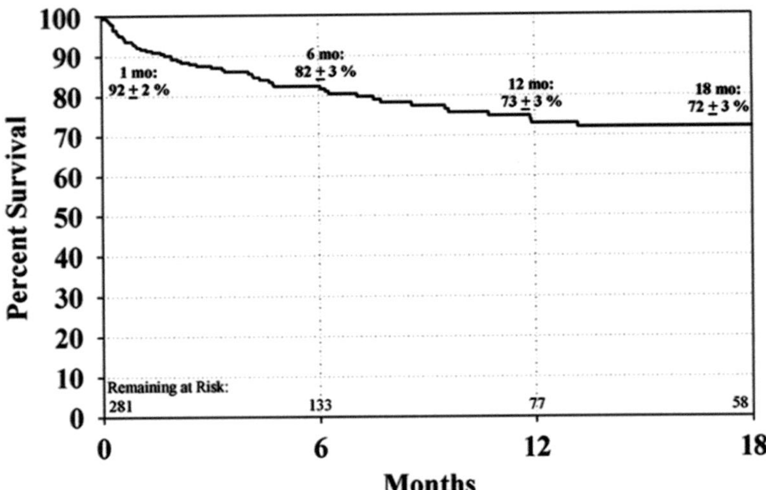

Fig. 2.3 Kaplan–Meier survival curve of continuous-flow LVAD [12]

with no valves or chambers. The most commonly used device worldwide, the HeartMate II, is an axial flow design with a rotor in the blood flow path suspended by bearings. The HeartMate II experience includes over 13,000 implantations. The HeartMate II began development in 1991 [9] with its first human implant in 2000. It has only one moving part, the rotor, which is suspended in the blood flow path by ruby bearings which, with in excess of eight-year follow-up, have yet to show significant bearing wear. Its speed typically ranges from 8,000 to 12,000 rpm, generating from 3 to 10 L/min of blood flow. It received Conformité Européenne Mark in November 2005, following its phase I trial, where patients improved their NYHA class as well as 60 % walked greater than 200 m than baseline [10], and received both BTT approval in 2008 and DT approval in 2010 by the US FDA.

2.4.2.1 Bridge to Transplantation

The HeartMate II received BTT approval based on the study published by Miller et al., in which 133 patients were implanted with the HeartMate II and followed them for 180 days [11]. This study found that at 3 months, there was significant improvement in functional status based on NYHA classification (80 % NYHA Class I or II), 6-min walk distance (increase threefold that of CRT), and quality of life based on questionnaires, both Minnesota Living with Heart Failure Questionnaire and Kansas City Cardiomyopathy Questionnaire. The survival rate was 75 % at 6 months and 68 % at 12 months. A follow-up study published by Pagani et al. in 2009 had further survival of 72 % at 18 months, [12] with 79 % either surviving, receiving transplantation, or having recovered and been explanted (Fig. 2.3). There was 92 % survival from any major device malfunction, which was a significant

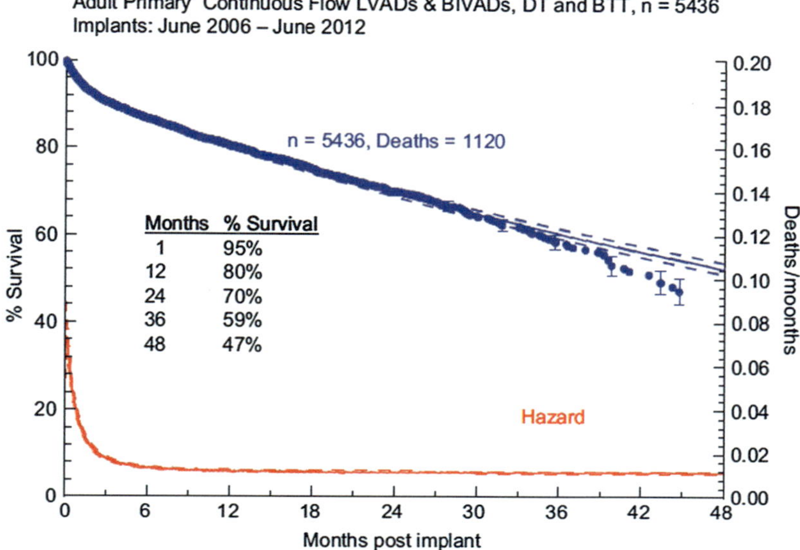

Fig. 2.4 INTERMACS actuarial survival for continuous-flow VADs (DT and BTT) [13]

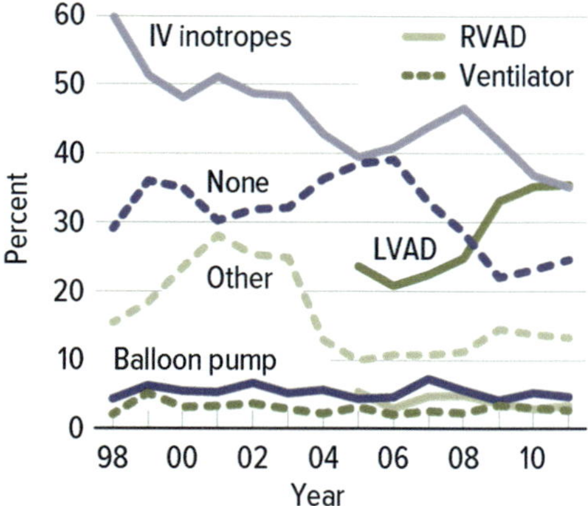

Fig. 2.5 Circulatory support prior to transplant [6]

improvement compared to the first-generation pulsatile devices. Most deaths occurred within the first 3 months and were attributable to stroke, infection, or multiorgan failure. Further post-approval data have shown survival at 12 months to be 80 % [13] (Fig. 2.4). These trials and any postanalysis have shown the HeartMate II to be effective at improving patient survival and quality of life while awaiting transplantation. The application of this technology is such that nearly 40 % of all recipients of donor heart receive a BTT VAD before transplant in the USA [6] (Fig. 2.5).

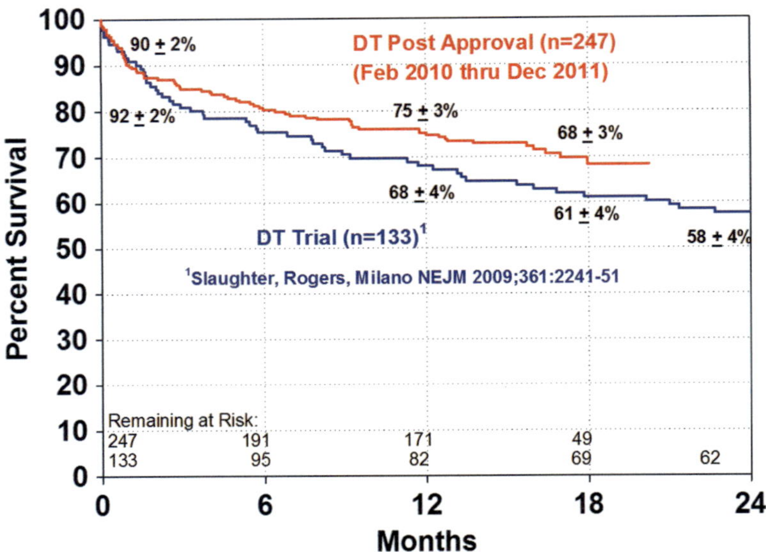

Fig. 2.6 Post-approval DT survival rates [15]

2.4.2.2 Destination Therapy

The HeartMate II received DT approval in 2010 in the USA based on the trial published by Slaughter et al. in 2009 [14]. This trial compared the HeartMate XVE to the HeartMate II in patients who were not considered transplant eligible. At the end of 2 years, 46 % of the patients with the HeartMate II had reached the primary endpoint versus 11 % of the patients with the HeartMate XVE. In addition, survival rates at 1 year and 2 years for patients with the HeartMate II were 68 % and 58 %, respectively, compared to 55 % and 24 % with the HeartMate XVE. These were significant advantages for the HeartMate II, which triggered its approval for DT. In post-approval analysis, as a result of improved knowledge of patient care nuances and less moribund recipient selection (see below), there has been improvement in survival of patients with 1-year survival to 75 % and 18-month survival of 68 % [15] (Fig. 2.6). At 2 years, the survival following DT VAD implantation approximates that of heart transplantation at 80 % [16].

2.4.3 Continuous-Flow Centrifugal Pumps

A new design model for continuous-flow LVAD is the centrifugal flow pumps, which also have levitation of the rotor, either through hydrodynamic forces or magnetic forces, or even both. The working idea is that this levitation may cause less wear on the device as well as provide wider gaps in the blood interface leading to less trauma to any blood cells, although explantation of the HeartMate II has shown minimal wear of the device with an expected device longevity of greater than 10 years [17]. The other advantage of these centrifugal pumps is that it can be smaller than the axial flow pumps and can be implanted directly in the pericardial cavity, whereas the HeartMate II implanted in the abdomen. Examples of these devices include the HeartMate III (Thoratec), the DuraHeart LVAS (Terumo), and the HVAD (Heartware). HVAD is the only device to receive formal BTT US approval, although the FDA has persistent unresolved concerns about the higher perioperative neurological events as well as the seven device failures. The HVAD was approved based on the ADVANCE-BTT trial, which compared 140 patients implanted with the HVAD in a study of non-inferiority to 499 control patients who were pooled from the INTERMACS registry after already receiving an FDA-approved VAD, most commonly the HeartMate II. The patients were followed for 180 days. The patient profiles were similar, except INTERMACS score suggested a more advanced population in the control arm, being 3.1 ± 1.3 in the HVAD arm and 2.7 ± 1.3 ($p < 0.01$) with 44.3 % of the HVAD arm being INTERMACS 3 (stable inotrope dependent) while the control group 51.9 % were profiled as INTERMACS 2 (unstable despite inotropes, vasoactive drugs, or intra-aortic balloon pump) (Table 2.2).

Table 2.2 Intermacs classifications [18]

Intermacs profile	Description	Time frame for intervention
Profile 1: critical cardiogenic shock	Patients with life-threatening hypotension despite rapidly escalating inotropic support, critical organ hypoperfusion, often confirmed by worsening acidosis and/or lactate levels	Definitive intervention needed within hours
Profile 2: progressive decline	Patient with declining function despite intravenous inotropic support may be manifest by worsening renal function, nutritional depletion, and inability to restore volume balance. Also describes declining status in patients unable to tolerate inotropic therapy	Definitive intervention needed within few days
Profile 3: stable but inotrope dependent	Patient with stable blood pressure, organ function, nutrition, and symptoms on continuous intravenous inotropic support (or a temporary circulatory support device or both), but of weeks to few months. N Demonstrating repeated failure to wean from support due to recurrent symptomatic hypotension or renal dysfunction	Definitive intervention elective over a period of weeks to few months
Profile 4: resting symptoms	Patient can be stabilized close to normal volume status but experiences daily symptoms of congestion at rest or during ADL. Doses of diuretics generally fluctuate at very high levels. More intensive management and surveillance strategies should be considered, which may in some cases reveal poor compliance that would compromise outcomes with any therapy. Some patients may alternate between 4 and 5	Definitive intervention elective over period of weeks to few months

(continued)

Table 2.2 (continued)

Intermacs profile	Description	Time frame for intervention
Profile 5: exertion intolerant	Comfortable at rest and with ADL but unable to engage in any other activity, living predominantly within the house. Patients are comfortable at rest without congestive nutrition, organ function, and activity. Symptoms, but may have underlying refractory elevated volume status, often with renal dysfunction. If underlying nutritional status and organ function are marginal, patient may be more at risk than INTERMACS 4 and require definitive intervention	Variable urgency, depends upon maintenance of nutrition, organ function, and activity
Profile 6: exertion limited	Patient without evidence of fluid overload is comfortable at rest and with activities of daily living and minor activities outside the home but fatigues after the first few minutes of any meaningful activity. Attribution to cardiac limitation requires careful measurement of peak oxygen consumption, in some cases with hemodynamic monitoring to confirm severity of cardiac impairment	Variable, depends upon maintenance of nutrition, organ function, and activity level
Profile 7: advanced NYHA III	A placeholder for more precise specification in future, this level includes patients who are without current or recent episodes of unstable fluid balance, living comfortably with meaningful activity limited to mild physical exertion	Transplantation or circulatory support may not currently be indicated

The primary endpoint of non-inferiority was met with an overall rate of 90.7 % in the HVAD arm being alive or transplanted compared to 90.2 % in the control arm. Only 21 % of the patients were transplanted within the 180-day trial window. In the study, there were 7 ischemic strokes in the HVAD arm, with the majority of these occurring within the first 2 days after implantation [19].

2.5 Patient Care

2.5.1 *Complications*

2.5.1.1 Thromboembolic Events

One of the initial concerns with the VAD was concern for excessive frequency of thrombosis and embolic events due to pump thrombosis and is the reason that patients with continuous-flow devices are placed on anticoagulation therapy with warfarin and antiplatelet therapy with aspirin. However, data from HeartMate II device has shown a relatively low number of ischemic strokes of 0.05 events per patient year (eppy), which is similar to patients with congestive heart failure and atrial fibrillation without a device [20]. As mentioned above, there is some concern with the HVAD in that it had an ischemic stroke rate of 0.12 eppy. Overall, the ischemic stroke rate is relatively low. Hemorrhagic strokes, which are uniformly fatal in this population, occur at a rate of 0.03 eppy for the HeartMate II and 0.07 eppy for the HVAD [19].

2.5.1.2   Infections

As all devices currently require external power, all devices have a driveline which penetrates the skin. This driveline is a nidus for infection and a serious concern. Driveline infection rates in the HeartMate II CAP study was 0.27 eppy and sepsis reported at 0.27 eppy [20]. Data suggest ischemic strokes and other complications may be associated with driveline infections. The HVAD had driveline infections of 0.25 eppy with sepsis in 0.23 eppy [19], so the persistence of infection will continue until there is a way to eliminate the driveline and transmit power wirelessly.

2.5.1.3   Gastrointestinal Bleeding

The continuous-flow devices currently have minimal pulsatility with their constant flow through the pump. In addition, the shear forces generated by all continuous-flow pumps (centrifugal or axial) uniformly result in cleaving of the von Willebrand factor yielding an acquired bleeding disorder or dual anticoagulation. This lack of pulsatility has also been associated with a significant increase in gastrointestinal bleeding compared to older pumps at a rate of 63 per 100 patient-years versus 6.8 per 100 patient-years for non-pulsatile versus pulsatile devices, respectively [21]. The bleeding has been typically an increase of micro-arteriovenous malformations, similar to that seen in patients with aortic stenosis (Heyde's syndrome). Despite the increase in bleeding with non-pulsatile devices versus pulsatile, there was no increase in mortality [21] suggesting these bleeds, while requiring transfusions, are not likely to result in mortality due to acute blood loss.

2.5.2   *Quality of Life*

All studies assessing quality of life (QoL) have shown significant improvement after patients receive a VAD, whether applying NYHA class, questionnaires, or 6-minute walk distances. In the HeartMate II DT trial, all patients were either NYHA Class IV or IIIb. At 6 months, 82 % were at NYHA Class I or II, and this persisted for the 24 months studied [20]. Six-minute walk distance increased from 214 to 372 m [20] (Fig. 2.7). Both the Kansas City Cardiomyopathy Questionnaire and the Minnesota Living with Heart Failure Questionnaire have shown positive results starting at 1 month and continuing to 6 months where there was a 47 % improvement in the

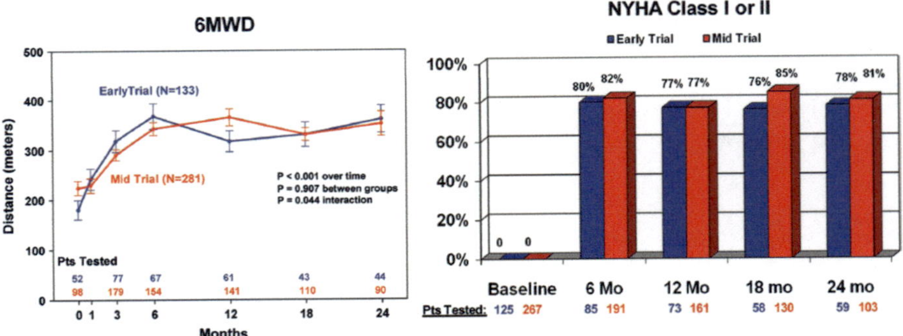

Fig. 2.7 Improvement in both 6-minute walk distance and NYHA class over time [20]

MLHF score from a baseline score of 71 to a 6-month score of 38 (lower score is better), and a 103 % improvement in KCCQ from baseline score of 31 to a 6-month score of 61 (higher score is better) [12].

2.6 Acceptance of Therapy

As a consequence of these excellent results, the application of this therapy has grown exponentially. Worldwide the number of annual HeartMate II implants has grown from approximately 1,900 in 2007 to 5,450 in 2012, almost threefold in 5 years. In the USSA, this was accounted for almost exclusively by the growth of DT since the number of BTT has remained relatively constant. In fact, since 2010, there have been significantly more DT than BTT implants: in 2012 approximately 2,350 BTT and 3,500 DT implants (50 % more DT).

2.6.1 Patient Selection

As implanting centers have become more knowledgeable about LVAD implantation and care, it has been discovered that waiting until patients are in cardiogenic shock, INTERMACS 1, prior to implantation, is associated with poor outcomes and these implants may be futile. In fact, the current trend when a patient is in critical cardiogenic shock is to stabilize the patient first with a short-term device such as a Tandem Heart or CentriMag (becoming the therapy of choice) or adding extracorporeal membrane oxygenation (ECMO) as a bridge to a BTT or DT durable VAD. The outcomes are far superior when a stable patient receives a durable VAD. Patients who were INTERMACS 1 had longer hospital stays post-implant and had worse survival compared to healthier patients. Patients dependent on inotropes, INTERMACS 2 and 3, also have increased mortality and length of stay compared to

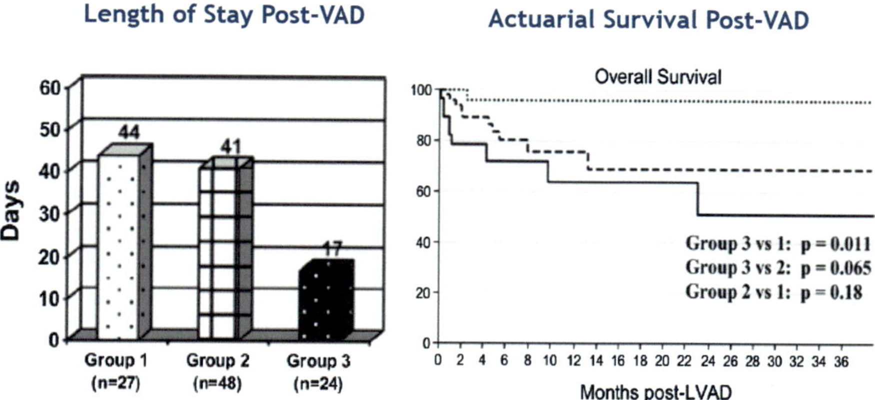

Fig. 2.8 Length of stay and survival based on pre-VAD INTERMACS classification [22]

healthier patients (INTERMACS 4–7) [22] (Fig. 2.8). As physicians have realized the benefits of LVAD therapy, and realizing that sicker patients do poorer, there has been a trend to implanting patients earlier. In 2007, 45.2 % of the implants were INTERMACS 1 while only 16.9 % were INTERMACS 3 and 4; in 2010 12.3 % of implants were INTERMACS 1, and 39.2 % were INTERMACS 3 and 4 [23]. However, disappointingly less than 20 % are INTERMACS 4–6, the severely limited group who are not on inotropes and who have the best survival at lowest cost. At the present time, Thoratec is conducting **R**isk Assessment and Comparative Assessment **O**f Left Ventricular **A**ssist **D**evice and **M**edical Management in **A**mbulatory Heart Failure **P**atients (ROADMAP), an observational study of INTERMACS 4–6 patients and will compare outcomes in those with implantation of the HeartMate II to optimal medical therapy, and is estimated to be completed in December 2015. In addition as a cooperative effort of the National Institutes of Health and Thoratec, the **R**andomized **E**valuation of **V**AD Intervention Before **I**notropic **T**herapy (REVIVE-IT) trial will randomize 100 NYHA class III patients (INTERMACS 6 and 7) to continued medical therapy or the HeartMate II and analyze outcomes. The outcomes of these studies may move the application of VADs into a less sick population.

2.6.2   *Implanting Centers*

2.6.2.1   Growth

As patient survival has improved with more modern devices as well as centers becoming more familiar with VAD implantation and care, the growth, especially in larger centers, has become almost exponential. In 2008, there were no centers that were managing 45 or more patients. In 2012, there are 28 centers, with seven managing 85 or more patients. As these centers continue to grow volume, they will have increased demand for nursing care, especially the care that VAD coordinators provide. Current suggested recommendations are that one VAD coordinator can safely manage no more than 15 VAD patients. With this current model, these large centers need six VAD coordinators, assuming no growth, which is not suggested based on prior trends. One potential solution to this model is the idea of shared care, or "hub and spoke" model.

With shared care, smaller satellite referral centers, or "spokes," will manage the patients on the majority of the routine follow-up with the patients with the dominant hospital, the "hub," seeing the patients intermittently, but always available to assist the smaller centers. As the smaller spokes become more comfortable managing the patients in their follow-up care, they may wish to consider becoming an implanting center for VAD, but still using the central hub hospital for transplants and other advanced or experimental therapies for heart failure. This model will spread the need of coordinators across a wider area, which would lessen the demand in each individual city.

2.6.2.2 Implantation at Non-transplant Open Heart Centers

One other advantage of the hub and spoke model of implanting centers is that centers can be closer to patient populations who have heart failure. Originally, implanting centers were only transplant centers (TC), and these were predominantly in metropolitan areas, and in the USA, these centers were predominantly in the northeastern region of the nation. The southern states, which have the highest incidence of heart failure deaths, have the fewest implanting centers. By enabling non-transplant open heart centers (OHC) to perform implants, patients will have easier access to this valuable technology. One fear of the larger hub centers is that these OHCs will implant only the low-risk population, leaving the high-risk patients for the hub center. This has not been proven in current experience. In a review of seventy-three patients implanted at OHC compared to 2,800 implanted at transplant centers, the patients implanted at the OHC were older, with 63 % at the OHC being greater than 60 compared to 42 % at the TC. 45 % were INTERMACS 1 or 2 at the OHC, compared to 56 % at the TC being INTERMACS 1 or 2. Overall survival was similar, with 1-year survival being $82\pm6\%$ at the OHC compared to 84 ± 1 % at the TC [24]. Overall in 2012, 389 of the implants were performed in OHCs. By partnering with these open heart centers, transplant centers can obtain access to patients that would not have been in their traditional catchment area.

2.7 The Team Approach to Care

In order to accommodate the growing patient volumes and access patients earlier in the course of their illness, comprehensive HF programs have evolved. These programs provide care for HF at all stages and include hospital to home transition programs, home telemonitoring, chronic disease management, and formal educational programs for patients and caregivers and AHF care including MCS and transplant. There are no longer "VAD" programs but "HF" programs that implant VADs as a form of therapy. This model allows access to MCS earlier in the disease process when the prognosis is better for a favorable outcome after implant and facilitates the care by the utilization of multidisciplinary teams.

The initial organizational difference includes the key role for the cardiologist who specializes in AHF. The American Board of Internal Medicine has recognized this key role by offering board certification in "Advanced Heart Failure and Transplant Cardiology" to board certified cardiologists who either have become expert in the management of HF by experience or training in Accreditation Council in Graduate Medical Education (ACGME)-approved fellowships. These cardiologists partner with the cardiac surgeon and are responsible of screening patients with AHF to determine their candidacy for implantation, chairing, or co-chairing the required committee which discusses each candidate, optimizing hemodynamics prior to implant to avoid RV failure and end-organ hypoperfusion injury, following the patient with the surgeon in the postoperative period, and providing and coordinating the long-term follow-up with the community cardiologist in the spoke. The partnership between the cardiologist and the surgeon is in part responsible for the superb outcomes and consistent growth of the application of this technology.

MCS lends itself to multidisciplinary care which includes but is not limited to VAD coordinators, nurse practitioners who provide the routine care, social service, palliative care, psychology, financial counseling, nutrition, and exercise physiology. In addition, medical specialists that need to contribute on the team are cardiac anesthesia, intensivists and hospitalists, pulmonology, gastroenterology, hematology, neurology, and nephrology.

2.8   Future Technologic Advances

The future for MCS is truly bright. Full magnetic levitation, as seen in the now defunct Levacor device which did not cleave the von Willebrand factor, is on the immediate horizon in the HeartMate III, a small profile centrifugal flow pump with full magnetic levitation which is entering into clinical trials in Europe in Fall 2013. Hopefully, the intensity of anticoagulation may also be safely reduced. This device will include pulsatility (30 min), which, in theory, will improve aortic root hemodynamics and may reduce the development of AV malformations in the gut. The next major innovation will be full implantability, the Fully Implantable Ventricular Assist System (FILVAS) of Thoratec which is being designed for the HeartMate II and HeartMate III and will utilize a small combined battery and system controller with a circumferential antenna for reception of a WiTricity signal to recharge the battery remotely from distance anticipated to be feet from the skin surface. This full implantability will eliminate driveline infections. Finally, the HeartMate X, as miniaturized version of axial flow technology, will be implanted with a minimally invasive technique and could be used in both RV and LV. In addition, this full support device will be weanable to 1 L/min flow to allow enhanced recovery by gradual reintroduction of preload and afterload. In fact, if the HeartMate II lasts the ten years that is predicted, the device exchange will incorporate minimally invasive, full magnetic levitation, pulsatility, and weanability all within the next decade.

2.9 Conclusions

Left ventricular assist devices have gone through significant changes since the original pneumatic pulsatile paracorporeal devices to current durable continuous-flow devices. These devices have enabled patients with AHF to have increased chance of long-term survival as well as vastly improved quality of life. As the growth of VADs continues to grow exponentially, new paradigms of care to provide access to a wider selection of patients have maturation, which include the hub and spoke model of a central transplant center and satellite smaller non-transplant implanting centers.

References

1. Braunwald E. Heart failure. JACC Heart Fail. 2013;1(1):1–20. doi:10.1016/j.jchf.2012.10.002.
2. Shiba N, Shimokawa H. Chronic heart failure in Japan: implications of the CHART studies. Vasc Health Risk Manag. 2008;4(1):103–13.
3. Hunt SA, Abraham WT, Chin MH, Feldman AM, Francis GS, Ganiats TG, et al. 2009 Focused update incorporated into the ACC/AHA 2005 guidelines for the diagnosis and management of heart failure in adults: a report of the American College of Cardiology Foundation/American Heart Association Task Force on Practice Guidelines: developed in collaboration with the international society for heart and lung transplantation. Circulation. 2009;119(14):e391–479. doi:10.1161/CIRCULATIONAHA.109.192065.
4. Cleland JGF, Clark AL. Delivering the cumulative benefits of triple therapy to improve outcomes in heart failure. J Am Coll Cardiol. 2003;42(7):1234–7. doi:10.1016/s0735-1097 (03)00948-3.
5. Metra M, Ponikowski P, Dickstein K, McMurray JJ, Gavazzi A, Bergh CH, Fraser AG, Jaarsma T, Pitsis A, Mohacsi P, Bohm M, Anker S, Dargie H, Brutsaert D, Komajda M. Heart failure association of the european society of c. advanced chronic heart failure: a position statement from the study group on advanced heart failure of the heart failure association of the european society of cardiology. Eur J Heart Fail. 2007;9(6–7):684–94. doi:10.1016/j.ejheart.2007.04.003.
6. OPTN/SRTR. Organ procurement and transplantation network (OPTN) and scientific registry of transplant recipients (SRTR). 2011 Annual data report. Department of Health and Human Services Health Resources and Services Administration, Healthcare systems Bureau, Division of Transplantation; 2012. http://optn.transplant.hrsa.gov/latestData/rptData.asp. Accessed 21 April 2012.
7. Boyle AJ. State of the state: opportunities and challenges today in VAD therapy. In: Presentation done at 2013 thoratec mechanical circulatory support (MCS) conference, Orlando, 2013.
8. Rose EA, Gelijns AC, Moskowitz AJ, Heitjan DF, Stevenson LW, Dembitsky W, Long JW, Ascheim DD, Tierney AR, Levitan RG, Watson JT, Ronan NS, Shapiro PA, Lazar RM, Miller LW, Gupta L, Frazier OH, Desvigne-Nickens P, Oz MC, Poirier VL, Meier P. Long-term use of a left ventricular assist device for end-stage heart failure. N Engl J Med. 2001;345(20):1435–43. doi: 10.1056/NEJMoa012175.

9. Griffith BP, Kormos RL, Borovetz HS, Litwak K, Antaki JF, Poirier VL, et al. HeartMate II left ventricular assist system: from concept to first clinical use. Ann Thorac Surg. 2001;71(90030):S116–20.

10. Kormos RL, Teuteberg JJ, Pagani FD, Russell SD, John R, Miller LW, et al. Right ventricular failure in patients with the HeartMate II continuous-flow left ventricular assist device: incidence, risk factors, and effect on outcomes. J Thorac Cardiovasc Surg. 2010;139(5):1316–24.

11. Miller LW, Pagani FD, Russell SD, John R, Boyle AJ, Aaronson KD, Conte JV, Naka Y, Mancini D, Delgado RM, MacGillivray TE, Farrar DJ, Frazier OH. Use of a continuous-flow device in patients awaiting heart transplantation. N Engl J Med. 2007;357(9):885–96. doi: 10.1056/NEJMoa067758.

12. Pagani FD, Miller LW, Russell SD, Aaronson KD, John R, Boyle AJ, et al. Extended mechanical circulatory support with a continuous-flow rotary left ventricular assist device. J Am Coll Cardiol. 2009;54(4):312–21. doi:10.1016/j.jacc.2009.03.055.

13. Kirklin JK, Naftel DC, Kormos RL, Stevenson LW, Pagani FD, Miller MA, et al. Fifth INTERMACS annual report: risk factor analysis from more than 6,000 mechanical circulatory support patients. J Heart Lung Transplant. 2013;32(2):141–56. doi:10.1016/j.healun.2012.12.004.

14. Slaughter MS, Rogers JG, Milano CA, Russell SD, Conte JV, Feldman D, Sun B, Tatooles AJ, Delgado RM, Long JW, Wozniak TC, Ghumman W, Farrar DJ, Frazier OH. Advanced heart failure treated with continuous-flow left ventricular assist device. N Engl J Med. 2009;361(23):2241–51. doi: 10.1056/NEJMoa0909938.

15. Jorde UP, Kushwaha SS, Tatooles AJ, Naka Y, Bhat G, Long JW, et al. 1 Initial results of the destination therapy post-FDA-approval study with a continuous flow left ventricular assist device: a prospective study using the INTERMACS registry. J Heart Lung Transplant. 2012;31(4):S10.

16. Kirklin JK, Naftel DC, Pagani FD, Kormos RL, Stevenson L, Miller M, et al. Long-term mechanical circulatory support (destination therapy): on track to compete with heart transplantation? J Thorac Cardiovasc Surg. 2012;144(3):584–603. doi:10.1016/j.jtcvs.2012.05.044.

17. Garbade J, Bittner HB, Barten MJ, Mohr FW. Current trends in implantable left ventricular assist devices. Cardiol Res Pract. 2011;2011:290561. doi: 10.4061/2011/290561.

18. Feldman D, Pamboukian SV, Teuteberg JJ, Birks E, Lietz K, Moore SA, et al. The 2013 international society for heart and lung transplantation guidelines for mechanical circulatory support: executive summary. J Heart Lung Transplant. 2013;32(2):157–87. doi:10.1016/j.healun.2012.09.013.

19. Godshall D. HeartWare® Ventricular Assist Device (HVAD®) circulatory systems device panel. 2012. http://www.fda.gov/downloads/AdvisoryCommittees/CommitteesMeetingMaterials/MedicalDevices/MedicalDevicesAdvisoryCommittee/CirculatorySystemDevicesPanel/UCM302187.pdf. Accessed 21 April 2013.

20. Park SJ, Milano CA, Tatooles AJ, Rogers JG, Adamson RM, Steidley DE, et al. Outcomes in advanced heart failure patients with left ventricular assist devices for destination therapy. Circ Heart Fail. 2012;5(2):241–8. doi:10.1161/CIRCHEARTFAILURE.111.963991.

21. Crow S, John R, Boyle A, Shumway S, Liao K, Colvin-Adams M, et al. Gastrointestinal bleeding rates in recipients of nonpulsatile and pulsatile left ventricular assist devices. J Thorac Cardiovasc Surg. 2009;137(1):208–15. doi:10.1016/j.jtcvs.2008.07.032.

22. Boyle AJ, Ascheim DD, Russo MJ, Kormos RL, John R, Naka Y, et al. Clinical outcomes for continuous-flow left ventricular assist device patients stratified by pre-operative INTERMACS classification. J Heart Lung Transplant. 2011;30(4):402–7.

23. Kirklin JK, Naftel DC, Kormos RL, Stevenson LW, Pagani FD, Miller MA, et al. The Fourth INTERMACS Annual Report: 4,000 implants and counting. J Heart Lung Transplant. 2012;31(2):117–26. doi:10.1016/j.healun.2011.12.001.

24. Katz MR, Horn EM, Dickinson MG, Zeevi GR, Salemi A, Slater JP. 4 Outcomes of patients implanted with a left ventricular assist device at non-transplant open heart surgery centers. J Heart Lung Transplant. 2012;31(4):S11.

Chapter 3
Older Destination Therapy Patient Selection

Robert M. Adamson and Walter P. Dembitksy

Abstract Portions of this chapter were presented at the 29th Annual Meeting and Scientific Sessions of the International Society for Heart and Lung Transplantation, April 2009, Paris, France and the 31st Annual Meeting and Scientific Sessions of the International Society for Heart and Lung Transplantation, April 2011, San Diego, California, USA. The abovementioned abstracts were published by Adamson et al. (J Am Coll Cardiol. 57(25):2487–95, 2011).

Keywords Destination therapy • Left ventricular assist devices (LVAD) • Older patients

3.1 Introduction

The utility and application of mechanical circulatory support (MCS) in patients with advanced heart failure has significantly progressed since the REMATCH trial demonstrated superiority of the HeartMate I left ventricular assist device (LVAD) over optimal medical management [1]. But these first-generation pulsatile devices were hindered by limited durability, high adverse event rates, and statistically significant but marginally improved survival rates over maximal medical management. Much of the reported literature on these first-generation devices identified older age as a risk factor for poor survival (Table 3.1) [2–17]. These studies have since become engrained into the prevailing clinical assumptions regarding the utility of mechanical support in the elderly. There are several aspects of these reports that make universal conclusions and inference from their findings suspect. Firstly, the studies could not agree on the age that imparted increased risk, varying from 49 to over 65

R.M. Adamson • W.P. Dembitksy (✉)
Sharp Memorial Hospital, San Diego, CA, USA
e-mail: dembitsky@aol.com

Table 3.1 Reported series on the impact of age on LVAD outcomes

References	Dates	Device	#	Indication	Criteria	Data type	Statistics
El-Banayosy et al. [2]	1992–2000	Thoratec	104	BTT	>60	Bad Oeynhausen	OR 3.87
Dang (2001)	1993–1999	Novacor	464	BTT	>65	Registry	OR 3.01
Granfeldt et al. [4]	1993–2003	Several	59	BTT		Sweden	NS
Rao et al. [11]	1996–2001	HMI	130	BTT	49±14	Columbia	NS
Dang et al. [5]	1996–2004	HMI	201	BTT	52±12	Columbia	1.89/10 years
Topkara et al. [16]	1996–2004	HMI	201		>60	Columbia	No change with age
Huang et al. [7]	1996–2003	Novacor	222		>60	Registry	OR 1.97
Schenk et al. [14]	1991–2002	Several	207		Older age	Cleveland	$P<04$
Holman et al. [6]	2006–2007	Several	420		50 vs. 60	INTERMACS	1.41
Sagrid (2009)	1998–2007	HMII	86	BTT	60	Vienna	Hazard 1.4
Schaffer et al. [13]	2000–2009	HMII	86	BTT	49±13	Johns Hopkins	1.07
Zahr (2009)	1991–2005	BiVAD	44	BTT			
Klotz et al. [9]	2003–2009	Several	241	BTT	>50	Muenster	OR 1.89
Leitz (2010)	1998–2005	HMI and II	377	DT		Registry	Center experience
Stepanenko et al. [15]	2006–2009	Several	28	DT	>65	Berlin	Significant
Kirklin et al. [8]	2006–2009	Several	1,092	Mixed	60–70	Registry	HR 2.42

years. The studies utilized first-generation devices which were no longer available due to poor outcome when compared with second-generation pumps. Much of the data was single center or registry data in origin with all of the inherently recognized shortcomings. There was also no differentiation on the indication for LVAD insertion; for example, failure to wean from cardiopulmonary bypass versus bridge to transplant or elective destination therapy was included without discrimination to outcome. Finally, outcomes associated with mechanical support have continued to improve in the current era due to better pumps, increased physician experience, and improved management protocols. Given these limitations, any assumptions regarding the survival disadvantage of supporting a patient over the age of 70 with the newer generation LVADs have to be reexamined in light of progress in the field.

A new era of MCS was ushered in by the development and subsequent FDA approval of the HeartMate II (HMII) continuous-flow LVAD [18–21]. With excellent durability, improved patient survival, decreased incidence of adverse events, and better patient satisfaction and quality of life, the HeartMate II was shown to be a superior option to the HeartMate I for both bridge to transplant (BTT) [18, 19] and destination therapy (DT) populations [20]. With an increasing population of elderly patients with advanced heart failure who have limited treatment options, there are unanswered questions pertaining to whether older patients can benefit from and are appropriate for this technology.

Congestive heart failure (CHF) is a common condition that increases with age. It is estimated that as many as 10 % of people over the age of 70 may be afflicted and as many as 150,000 experience class IV symptoms [22]. Medical management of this population is expensive and offers limited survival and potential for functional recovery. Cardiac transplantation has traditionally been the gold standard for comparing end-stage heart failure management but with a small donor pool (approximately 2,000 per year in the USA), and with the pragmatic restriction to patients under the age of 70 years, it appears that MCS will become the standard of care for older, refractory heart failure patients.

Patients with conditions such as advanced age, remote history of cancer, active infections, renal insufficiency, pulmonary artery hypertension, sensitization, and large body size especially with a common blood type could potentially be transplanted, but their waiting times are typically prolonged. Older patients ($\geq$70 years) are the largest potential group that could benefit from LVAD support, yet advanced age has consistently been identified as a risk factor for poor outcome. As noted above, these studies have several limitations: (1) use of proven inferior technology (pulsatile devices), (2) registry data of LVADs in patients with diverse indications (i.e., failure to wean from CBP, deterioration while awaiting transplantation, and ongoing cardiogenic shock), and (3) data from a variety of mixed low- and high-volume centers. Therefore, extrapolation from these earlier results may not accurately reflect the expected outcome with the newer continuous-flow HMII device. Hence, the main objective of our study [23] was to evaluate the outcomes of LVAD patients older than 70 years of age from a community hospital with an experienced VAD team.

3.2 Methods of Our Initial Evaluation of Elderly Compared to Younger Patients

3.2.1 Patient Inclusion Criteria

All patients studied met the clinical trial enrollment criteria and the general criteria for BTT/DT LVAD implantation as published by the Centers for Medicare and Medicaid Services (CMS) [23], including chronic end-stage heart failure (New York Heart Association [NYHA] class IV symptoms failing to respond to optimal medical management, end-stage left ventricular failure for at least 90 days, and a life expectancy of less than 2 years); left ventricular ejection fraction (LVEF) <25 %; demonstrated functional limitation with peak $VO_2 < 12$ mL/kg/min; or continued need for intravenous (I.V.) inotropic therapy; and an appropriate body size to support LVAD implantation [23].

3.2.2 Facility Criteria

Through a National Coverage Determination issued on October 2003, Medicare began coverage of the DT indication, and effective March 27, 2007, new facility criteria were established which require hospitals to receive certification from the Joint Commission on Accreditation of Healthcare Organizations (JCAHO) [23]. Facilities gaining JCAHO certification are placed on a list on the CMS website, which is continuously updated [23, 24]. During the current study, our facility achieved and maintained JCAHO certification as a Medicare-approved VAD facility.

3.2.3 Preoperative Assessment and Clinical Optimization

The criteria adopted for selecting LVAD candidates are summarized in Table 3.2. All patients underwent comprehensive evaluation and treatment prior to LVAD placement, which included clinical assessment of the severity of heart failure, hemodynamic state, cardiac anatomy, and operative risk. Inotropic support, diuresis or ultrafiltration, infection surveillance/treatment, and nutritional assistance were provided when needed. Based on the response to treatment, it was determined if the patient should continue on medical treatment or hospice and offered high-risk surgical repair with LVAD standby or become a candidate for destination LVAD therapy or transplantation. For nonresponders the decision was whether they were appropriate LVAD candidates or too sick for support. Noncardiac considerations such as history of chronic or life-limiting illnesses, mental status, nutritional status, expectations (quality of life vs. duration of life), and psychosocial and age-related considerations were assessed.

Table 3.2 Criteria for selecting patients as LVAD candidates

Characteristics of patients selected for LVAD therapy	High-risk LVAD patients but not absolute contraindicators	Contraindications to LVAD support
Intolerable congestive heart failure symptoms and/or lifestyle limitations despite maximal medical/surgical therapies	Severe chronic obstructive pulmonary disease (COPD)	Patient refusal
Meets national standardized inclusion criteria	History of stroke with worsened neurocognitive defect secondary to congestive heart failure	Insufficient significant other support, home environment, or financial resources
Adequate mental, psychological, social, and financial support to comply with the complex LVAD management protocols	Primary right heart failure (i.e., hypertrophic myopathy, arrhythmogenic right ventricular dysplasia, or posttransplant constrictive/restrictive disease)	Irreversible neurocognitive defects that preclude routine LVAD care
A strong desire to have an LVAD implanted held by both the patient and his significant other caregivers	Fixed pulmonary artery hypertension	Ongoing cardiogenic shock refractory to all resuscitation measures including peripheral cardiopulmonary bypass (CPB) resuscitation
	Active infections	End-stage pulmonary disease out of proportion to congestive heart failure
	Hepatic fibrosis or cirrhosis	Fungemia
	Blood dyscrasias (heparin-induced thrombocytopenia, hypercoagulable states, current 2B3A drug use)	Ongoing drug or alcohol addiction or recent history of noncompliance to medical therapy
	Renal failure including chronic dialysis dependence	
	Patient or significant other ambivalence regarding the LVAD implant	

Neurological Assessment A neurological evaluation was ordered if necessary to rule out degenerative central nervous system (CNS) diseases and dementia. Since it is imperative that candidates for LVAD therapy demonstrate the ability to operate the device safely, we assessed for stroke, psychiatric disorders, mental retardation, substance abuse, and other factors which could potentially impact compliance with medical regimen and clinic visit follow-ups [25].

Renal Assessment Patient's baseline renal function was reviewed since poor baseline renal function is associated with worse outcomes after LVAD implantation [26–28]. This included assessment of renal parameters as well as preoperative diuretics and aggressive treatment of heart failure (inotropic support, ultrafiltration, or dialysis).

Nutritional Assessment For each patient, a comprehensive assessment was made to define the degree of malnutrition and estimate the severity of illness (SI). The Subjective Global Assessment (SGA) and SI scales were typically used to determine the level of malnutrition and to determine when to start nutritional support [29].

Psychosocial Assessment When evaluating the patient's social support network, the following were reviewed: the presence and age of the caregiver, such as a spouse or family member, who could be available in case of device malfunction; a plan of care for discharge which would ensure that the home environment was safe and allow the patient to receive adequate postoperative care; and the patient's ability to care for himself, including eyesight, hearing, dexterity, and evidence of poor dentition, as well as any history of noncompliance with medical regimens. Social workers reviewed the availability of patient-related community resources. If significant questions were unanswered, then a trained home health nurse visited the patient's home to complete the assessment.

Informed Consent All patients received the information necessary to assist them in giving appropriate informed consent for the procedure. The patient and significant others signed a health-care contract delineating the expectations for aftercare.

Post-Op Management Prevention of right heart failure was implemented in all patients, which included the routine use of inhaled nitric oxide, bi-ventricular pacing when necessary, and the use of inotropic drugs, such as isoproterenol, dopamine, and milrinone in the immediate postoperative period. Patients with impaired right ventricular function were given sildenafil routinely and the inhaled nitric oxide was weaned within 24–48 h in most cases. Nursing care in the cardiac step-down unit focused on strengthening, self-care, and education about LVAD management.

3.2.4 Patient Population

In our initial study [30], 55 consecutive patients receiving HMII LVADs included in the BTT or DT clinical trials from October 2005 through January 2010 at a small community hospital with extensive MCS experience were evaluated. Patients were divided into two groups based on age at the time of implant: Group 1, patients under the age of 70 ($n=25$) and Group 2, patients 70 years or older ($n=30$). During the study period, 329 patients were referred for consideration of LVAD or transplantation of which 15 % (49/280) were 70 years or older. The majority of patients, 61 % (30/49), 70 years of age or older, accepted and underwent HMII implant. Four patients (8 %) were considered to be good candidates but refused our recommendation; 16 % (8/49) were too well while only 8 % (4/49) were too ill. In the younger than 70 population 46 % (103/280) either received a HMII or were transplanted, 14 % (40/280) were too well, 5 % (13/280) underwent a traditional cardiac operation, 4 % (10/280) were too ill, 13 % (37/280) were not considered to be good LVAD candidates, 8 % (24/280) failed to keep their appointment, and 3 % (9/280) refused to accept our advice for LVAD or transplant. Only patients implanted as part of the HMII trial were studied since complete datasets were available only for these patients.

3.2.5 Outcomes

The two groups were compared with regard to preoperative patient characteristics and outcome measures including Kaplan–Meier survival, prevalence and incidence of adverse events, quality of life metrics (Kansas City Cardiomyopathy Questionnaire [KCCQ], clinical summary score [CSS], and overall summary scores [OSS], Minnesota Living With Heart Failure Questionnaire [MLWHF]), and functional status six-minute walk distance [6MWD], New York Heart Association (NYHA) function class, and patient activity levels with Metabolic Equivalent Task Score (METS) [21].

3.2.6 Statistical Analysis

Statistical analyses except for Poisson regression were done using Systat (Cranes Software, Chicago, IL). Poisson regression was performed using SAS (SAS Institute Inc., Cary, NC). Differences between groups of independent, normally distributed, continuous variables were evaluated using the t-test. Variables that were not normally distributed were evaluated using the Mann–Whitney U-test. Normality was checked using the Anderson–Darling test. Differences in categorical variables were evaluated using the Fisher's exact test. Statistical comparisons were two-sided and the level of significance was set at $p < 0.05$. Survival analysis was performed using the Kaplan–Meier method with patients censored for transplantation, recovery of the native heart function with device removal, or withdrawal from the study. Comparison of survival between the two groups was performed using the log-rank test. Adverse events were presented as both percentages of patients and event rates (events per patient-year). Comparisons of adverse event rates between the two groups were performed using a Poisson regression model (Mantel–Haenszel), with the total duration of support as the exposure time and total number of events as the response variable. Quality of life comparisons were performed using linear mixed effects modeling (mixed subroutine in Systat). The predictor variables were age group and time group (baseline, 1, 3, and 6 months). Time group: Eight patients (four in each group) had a previous pulsatile flow LVAD which was replaced with a HMII LVAD. Duration of support and survival for these patients was evaluated from the date of the first LVAD implant. Only adverse events that were observed when on the HMII device were included.

3.3 Results

3.3.1 Baseline Patient Characteristics

The age distribution of LVAD patients in this study shows most who were between the ages of 60 and 80 (Fig. 3.1). Baseline characteristics were similar between groups except for age, nutritional status (prealbumin), use of ACE inhibitors, and

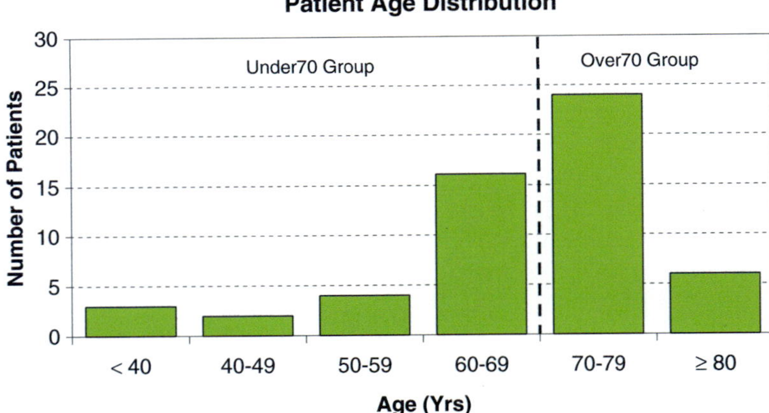

Fig. 3.1 Age distribution of patients evaluated in this study

ventilator support (Table 3.3). There was a tendency for a higher prevalence of ischemic etiologies and prior cardiac resynchronization therapy in the >70 age group compared to the <70 age group, but these differences were not statistically significant. All patients were in NYHA class IV prior to the LVAD implant. There was no difference in the mean Leitz–Miller destination therapy risk score [31] between the <70 (10.5±6.3) and >70 (8.3±5.8, $p=0.205$) groups, nor in the percentage of patients with high/very high-risk scores or low-risk scores.

3.3.2 Operative Procedures

Associated concomitant operative procedures are listed in Table 3.4. Four patients in each group had a prior HeartMate XVE exchanged for a HMII. There were no statistically significant differences between the two groups in the number of patients undergoing mitral valve repair/replacement, tricuspid valve repair/replacement, aortic valve patch closure, patent foramen ovale closure, or any other concomitant procedures performed at the time of surgery. One >70 patient had a right ventricular assist device (RVAD) [Biomedicus pump] which was removed after two days, while none in the <70 group. Cardiopulmonary bypass times were similar between the <70 and >70 groups (80±32 vs. 83±41 min, $p=0.760$).

3.3.3 Duration of Support

Patients in the <70 group were supported for an average of 678±676 days (median=415, range: 8 days–8 years), while patients in the >70 group were supported

Table 3.3 Baseline characteristics of patients used in the study. Body surface area (BSA), weight, cardiac index (CI), pulmonary capillary wedge pressure (PCWP), systolic blood pressure, albumin, prealbumin, and destination therapy risk score (DTRS) were normally distributed and evaluated using the t-test. The remaining continuous variables [left ventricular ejection fraction (LVEF), creatinine, blood urea nitrogen (BUN), alanine aminotransferase (ALT), aspartate aminotransferase (AST), total bilirubin (TBILI), sodium (NA)] were evaluated using the nonparametric Mann–Whitney U-test

| | Age group | | |
Parameter	Under 70 years ($n=25$)	Over 70 years ($n=30$)	P
Patients enrolled (%)	25 (45)	30 (55)	–
Age (years)	56.7 ± 14.3	76.3 ± 3.9	<0.001
[min–max]	[16–69]	[70–87]	
Ischemic (%)	15 (60)	24 (80)	0.140
BSA (m^2)	1.98 ± 0.21	1.95 ± 0.19	0.671
Weight (kg)	83 ± 15	79 ± 15	0.276
LVEF (%)	21 ± 9	20 ± 6	0.651
CI (L/min/m^2)	1.95 ± 0.72	1.67 ± 0.49	0.139
PCWP (mmHg)	27 ± 9	27 ± 9	0.824
Systolic BP (mmHg)	104 ± 19	108 ± 15	0.438
Creatinine (mg/dL)	1.76 ± 1.17	1.47 ± 0.61	0.420
BUN (mg/dL)	34.3 ± 20.1	32.8 ± 15.4	0.939
ALT (U/L)	81 ± 209	62 ± 123	0.205
AST (U/L)	98 ± 165	44 ± 48	0.141
TBILI (mg/dL)	1.08 ± 0.78	0.99 ± 0.53	0.932
Albumin (g/dL)	3.55 ± 0.52	3.76 ± 0.52	0.137
Prealbumin (mg/dL)	16 ± 7	21 ± 6	0.030
Na (mM/L)	135.3 ± 5.5	136.9 ± 4.6	0.297
Beta-blockers (%)	6 (24)	13 (43)	0.163
ACE inhibitors (%)	2 (8)	13 (43)	0.005
Intravenous inotrope agents (%)	17 (68)	18 (60)	0.585
Single inotrope (%)	10 (40)	14 (47)	0.785
More than one inotrope (%)	7 (28)	4 (13)	0.198
CRT (%)	9 (36)	19 (63)	0.06
ICD (%)	16 (64)	25 (83)	0.128
Ventilator support (%)	5 (20)	0 (0)	0.015
IABP (%)	3 (12)	0 (0)	0.088
DTRS	10.5 ± 6.3	8.3 ± 5.8	0.205
DTRS—Low risk (%)	10 (40)	15 (50)	0.588
DTRS—High/very high risk (%)	5 (20)	4 (13)	0.716

Table 3.4 Associated operative procedures

| | Age group (%) | | |
Procedure	Under 70 years ($n=5$)	Over 70 years ($n=30$)	P
XVE replaced with a HMII	4 (16)	4 (13)	1.000
Mitral valve repair/replacement	8 (32)	11 (37)	0.781
Tricuspid valve repair/replacement	5 (20)	5 (17)	1.000
Aortic valve patch closure	6 (24)	7 (23)	1.000
Patent foramen ovale closure	3 (12)	2 (7)	0.650
Other procedures	5 (20)	7 (23)	1.000

Other procedures include cardiopulmonary support removal, coronary artery bypass, hernia repair, right ventricle/left ventricular pacing lead placement, bronchoscopy, left atrial appendage ligation, and cryoablation

for 539 ± 475 (median$=482$ days, range: 19 days–5.6 years) ($p=0.630$). Thirteen patients in Group 1 were supported with an LVAD for >1 year, including nine patients >2 years, four patients >3 years, three patients >4 years, and the longest at 8 years. Comparatively, 16>70 patients were supported >1 year, including eight patients >2 years, four patients >3 years, two patients >4 years, and the longest 5.6 years.

3.3.4 Outcomes

The Kaplan–Meier survival rates for both groups were comparable (log-rank $p=0.806$) (Fig. 3.2a). Survival rates for <70 vs. >70 groups were similar at 30 days (96 % vs. 97 %), 6 months (88 % vs. 83 %), 1 year (72 % vs. 75 %), and 2 years (65 % vs. 70 %). Survival rates for patients receiving the HMII as their initial device, after excluding those who received it as an exchange for the XVE, were also similar ($p=0.898$) at 1 year (65 % vs. 70 %) and 2 years (65 % vs. 70 %) (Fig. 3.2b). In the <70 group, six patients (24 %) died, two patients (8 %) were transplanted, one patient (4 %) recovered cardiac function and had the LVAD removed, and 16 patients (64 %) were still ongoing LVAD support (3<1 year, 13>1 year) at 1 year. Similarly, in the >70 group, seven patients (23 %) died, none were transplanted or recovered cardiac function, and 23 (77 %) were still ongoing on LVAD support (7 patients <1 year, 16 patients >1year) at 1 year. No significant differences in the causes of death were observed between the two groups (Table 3.5).

3.3.5 Length of Stay and Hospital Course

The average length of stay in the hospital was similar for the <70 and >70 groups (23 ± 14 days vs. 24 ± 15 days, $p=0.805$). Some patients stayed longer in the ICU primarily for respiratory care and right ventricular weaning of intravenous inotropic medications. Non-device-related re-hospitalizations included infirmaries related to orthopedic surgery, cholecystectomy, transuretheral resection of the prostate, and *Clostridium difficile* infection.

3.3.6 Quality of Life and Functional Status

Outcomes associated with the quality of life and functional status are shown in Table 3.6. The percentage of patients in NYHA class I or II improved from 0 % at baseline to 100 % (<70 group) and 89 % (>70 group) at 6 months. There were statistically significant improvements in 6MWD distance from baseline (for those able to walk) to 6 months for <70 group (256–275 m) and >70 group (233–295 m). There

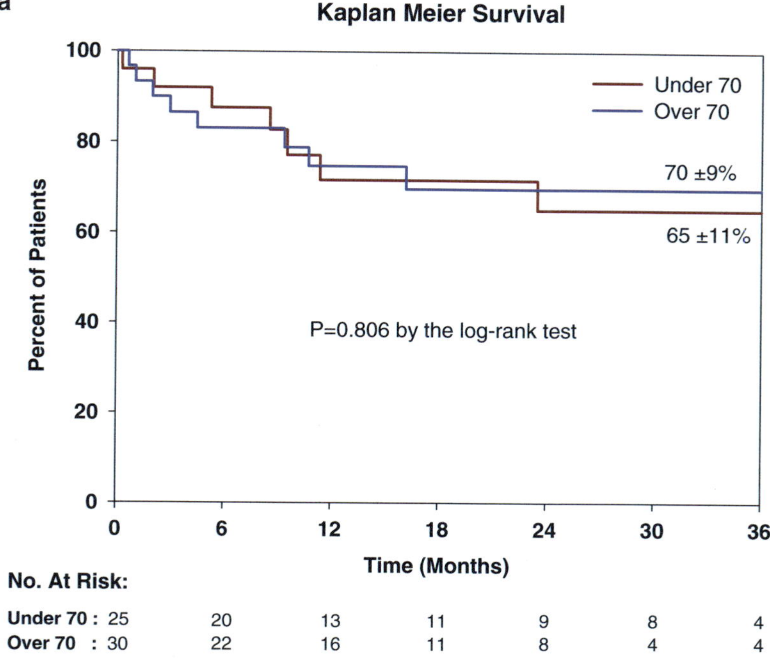

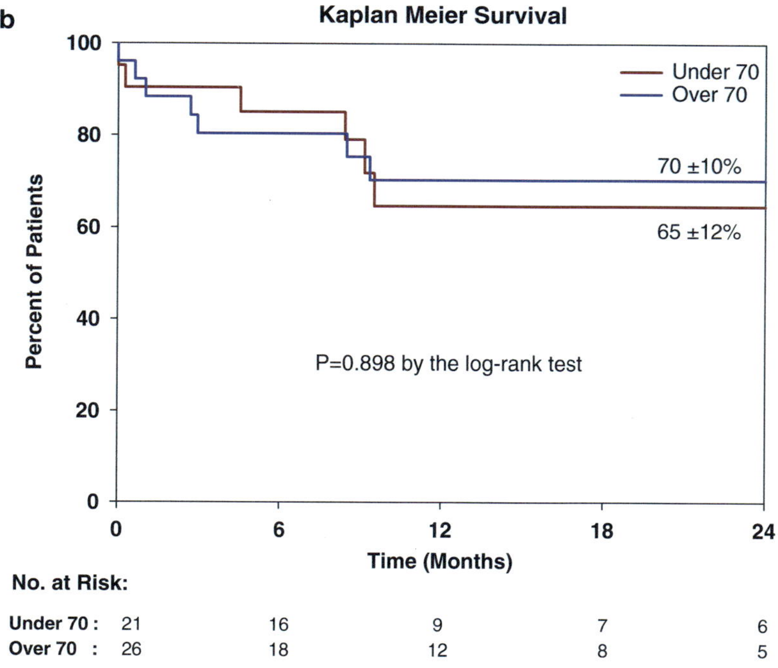

Fig. 3.2 (**a**) Kaplan–Meier survival curves including patients who had a HeartMate XVE replaced with a HMII. (**b**) Kaplan–Meier survival curves for patients with the HMII as their first device, excluding patients who had a HeartMate XVE replaced with a HMII

Table 3.5 Causes of death

	Percent of implanted patients (%)		
Cause of death ≤12 months	Under 70 years ($n=6/25$; 24 %)	Over 70 years ($n=7/30$; 23 %)	P
Sepsis	1 (4)	1 (3)	1.000
Respiratory failure	2 (8)	1 (3)	0.586
Multiorgan failure	0 (0)	1 (3)	1.000
Ischemic stroke	1 (4)	0 (0)	0.455
Hemorrhagic stroke	0 (0)	1 (3)	1.000
Device thrombosis	1 (4)	0 (0)	0.455
Patient disconnected power	1 (4)	0 (0)	0.455
Cancer	0 (0)	1 (3)	1.000
Withdrawal of support	0 (0)	1 (3)	1.000
Unknown	0	1 (3)	1.000
Causes of death > 12 months	Under 70 years ($n=2/25$; 8 %)	Over 70 years ($n=3/30$; 10 %)	
Anoxic brain injury	0 (0)	1 (3)	1.000
Cardiomyopathy	1 (4)	0 (0)	0.455
Sepsis	1 (4)	0 (0)	0.455
Unknown	0 (0)	1 (3)	1.000
Respiratory failure	0 (0)	1 (3)	1.000

were also significant improvements by approximately 36 (<70 group) and 42 points (>70 group) at 6 months in heart failure-related quality of life metrics using the Minnesota Living With Heart Failure Questionnaire. Similarly, there was a 32-point increase (<70 group) and a 42-point increase (>70 group) in mean values of the Kansas City Cardiomyopathy Questionnaire overall summary score (Table 3.6). Patient activity levels significantly increased in this period as well. The percent of patients achieving METS 3 (moderate activity) or higher improved from 12 % at baseline to 63 % at 6 months (<70 group) compared to 7–52 % (>70 group). Overall, there was no difference in any of the quality of life or functional status metrics between the two groups.

3.3.7 Adverse Events

The incidence of adverse events (Table 3.7) was similar between Group 1 (<70) and Group 2 (>70) for bleeding requiring PRBC (0.33 vs. 42 events/patient-year, $p=0.591$) and requiring surgery (0.15 vs. 0.11, $p=0.583$), device-related infection (0.15 vs. 0.13 events/patient-year, $p=0.813$), incidence of hemorrhagic (0.03 vs. 0.05 events/patient-year, $p=0.557$), and ischemic strokes (0.03 vs. 0.03 events/patient-year, $p=0.985$).

Table 3.6 Functional capacity and quality of life

	Under 70					Over 70					
	Baseline	1 month	3 months	6 months	P^a	Baseline	1 month	3 months	6 months	P^a	P^b
NYHA class											
Pts tested at interval	24	21	21	20		29	26	20	19		
Class I/II (%)	0 (0)	10 (48)	18 (86)	20 (100)	<0.001	0 (0)	11 (42)	18 (90)	17 (89)	<0.001	0.351
Six-minute walk test											
Pts tested at interval	6	14	18	17		15	17	17	15		
Distance walked (m)	256±96	188±113	354±162	275±135	<0.001	233±100	162±114	256±100	295±97	0.004	0.221
Minnesota Living With Heart Failure											
Pts tested at interval	18	20	22	20		26	23	20	17		
Score	73±33	65±26	41±23	37±26	<0.001	65±21	50±23	46±28	23±19	<0.001	0.072
Kansas City Cardiomyopathy Questionnaire											
Pts tested at interval	18	20	22	20		25	23	22	18		
Overall summary score	32±28	40±27	61±26	64±26	<0.001	33±18	42±23	60±24	75±24	<0.001	0.587
Clinical summary score	41±29	47±26	67±22	70±25	<0.001	42±19	45±22	63±20	77±21	<0.001	0.881
Patient activity levels (METS)											
Pts tested at interval	25	23	23	19		30	27	23	20		
% METS 3 or higher	3 (12)	4 (17)	15 (65)	12 (63)	<0.001	2 (7)	4 (15)	12 (52)	17 (85)	<0.001	0.205

[a]p value for changes over time
[b]p value for differences between older and younger patients

Table 3.7 Adverse events

Adverse events	Under 70 years ($n=25$) 38.8 pt. years		Over 70 years ($n=30$) 37.7 pt. years		
	Incidence pts (%)	Event rate (events/pt-year)	Incidence pts (%)	Event rate (events/pt-year)	P
Bleeding requiring PRBC	7 (28)	0.33	9 (30)	0.42	0.591
Bleeding requiring re-exploration	5 (20)	0.15	3 (10)	0.11	0.583
Infection					
Local non-device-related	12 (48)	0.67	14 (47)	0.72	0.853
Sepsis	6 (24)	0.21	6 (20)	0.19	0.854
Device-related	5 (20)	0.15	5 (17)	0.13	0.813
Cardiac arrhythmias: cardioversion/defibrillation	8 (32)	0.26	10 (33)	0.29	0.802
Renal failure	1 (4)	0.03	1 (3)	0.03	0.984
Right heart failure	1 (4)	0.03	1 (3)	0.03	0.984
RVAD	0 (0)	0.00	1 (3)	0.03	0.317
Ischemic stroke	1 (4)	0.03	1 (3)	0.03	0.984
Hemorrhagic stroke	1 (4)	0.03	2 (7)	0.05	0.557
Other neurological events (e.g., TIA, seizures, confusion)	4 (16)	0.10	3 (10)	0.08	0.746
Hemolysis	0 (0)	0.00	0 (0)	0.00	–

Patients older than 70 years of age receiving the HeartMate II left ventricular assist device: a community hospital experience

3.3.8 *More Recent Comparison of Patients > 70 Years to Younger Patients*

Results were then updated with comparison of all 152 patients undergoing HMII implant at our institution since 2005 to determine if age ≥ 70 predicted survival. Kaplan–Meier analysis determined statistical significance.

There is again no survival disadvantage when patients ≥ 70 years are compared to the younger cohort. Furthermore, when the most recent overall survival is compared to the earlier BTT and DT study cohorts, there is an improvement in survival for both groups (see Fig. 3.3).

3.4 Discussion

These studies show that excellent results can be obtained with LVAD support as destination therapy in advanced heart failure patients over age 70. We believe that this type of mechanical support should be considered as an attractive option for select patients refractory to maximal medical therapy and that age should not be an

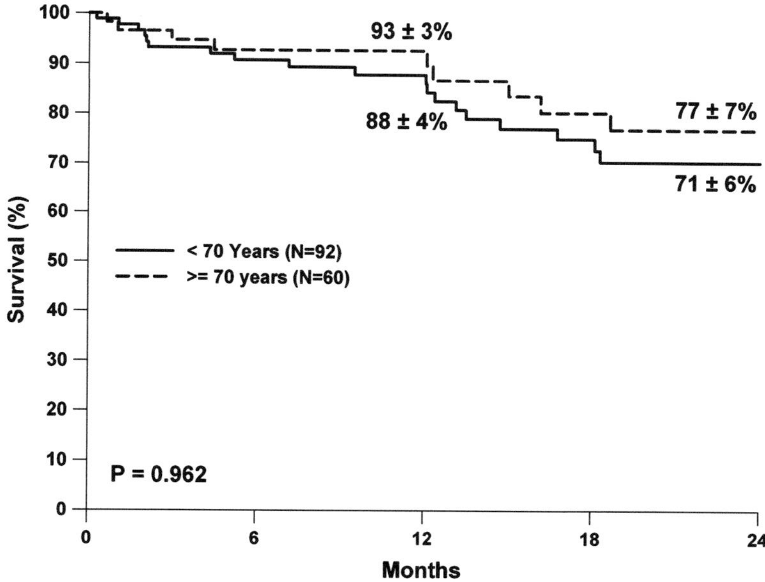

Fig. 3.3 Actuarial survival for patients receiving a HeartMate II LVAD analyzed by age, < 70 years compared to > 70 years

absolute contraindication to LVAD support. The results also indicate that very good results can be achieved in a community hospital setting with a focused effort from a dedicated team.

Despite the facts that heart failure is a major public health problem affecting more than five million Americans with an estimated 250,000 in class IV heart failure, and there was proven superiority with early LVAD technology over medical therapy, there was only a modest increase in the number of patients receiving LVADs. Lietz et al. reported that only 451 patients underwent DT device placement with pulsatile LVADs during the first 5 years after REMATCH, and DT accounted for only 17 % of the devices implanted [10]. Also, with the incidence of NYHA class IV heart failure increasing with age, one would expect national LVAD volumes to dramatically increase in elderly patients, but this has not been the case.

The main reason for this discrepancy is that the pulsatile devices had poor reliability and significant adverse events rates. Although there was a survival advantage demonstrated in REMATCH, the outcomes led many to question if the increased duration of life was worth the expense to both the patients and the health-care system. Age is another factor which has consistently been identified in multiple studies as a risk factor for decreased survival and increased adverse events after LVAD placement [2–17]. However, these previous studies have significant limitations. First, the impact of comorbidities and the presence of irreversible cardiogenic shock were not controlled. Second, many studies used a mixture of devices in their review, which may confound the overall analysis [20], and some of the data comes from registries where the robustness of the data is suspect. Given these shortcomings, we do not have sufficient published data on continuous-flow devices implanted at experienced centers to conclude that advanced age should be a contraindication to LVAD therapy.

One important positive factor in the use of LVAD therapy in older patients is that the patients are very appreciative of the improved quality of life afforded by the LVAD. While younger patients want to live longer, older patients want to live better. Older patients are also typically more compliant with medications and instructions from caregivers and do not have increased adverse events just because of their age. Older patients tend to be less active in general and seem to have fewer driveline-related complications. They often have support adult children that are willing to assist in the postoperative care. Additionally, many have achieved a degree of financial security that allows them the luxury of not needing to be employed, and their health-care benefits are not in jeopardy of being terminated.

There are some patient-specific precautions that coincide with advanced age. For example, their generalized poor eyesight and decreased manual dexterity require additional training and practice to assure safety in battery change. Their partners also tend to be older, and in fact, many older LVAD recipients are the primary caregivers for their spouses. Older patients have significantly more associated illnesses: prostate cancer, COPD, peripheral vascular disease, diabetes, and generalized debility making access to a rehabilitation support if necessary. They may also have a higher incidence of native valvular insufficiency in the aortic, mitral, and tricuspid positions. These may require repair at the time of initial LVAD insertion.

Selecting the right older patient is critical. Older patients can have more associated illnesses and other concomitant problems with the native heart that need to be considered. Rigorous assessment and optimization of preoperative status should be undertaken, including neurological, nutritional, psychosocial, and renal assessments. Optimal outcomes in LVAD patients can be achieved with a dedicated LVAD team organized and charged with implantation, early postoperative management, and outpatient management, as outlined in a recent publication on clinical management of continuous-flow LVADs [30]. Our study shows that if such practices are adopted, then good outcomes can be achieved.

Center experience has been shown to play an important role in determining outcomes with LVAD therapy [10]. Our implant techniques, patient selection, and management protocols are constantly improving. This study demonstrates that DT LVAD therapy can safely be delivered in a small community hospital with an experienced team in an older patient population. In fact, Sharp Hospital survival rates are higher and the rates of adverse events are lower in both groups when compared to the results of the multicenter HMII trials [18–20]. Similar outcomes can be achieved in other hospital settings as well.

Patient selection is an important question to be answered if these results are to be duplicated in other centers. The majority of referred patients >70 years of age (61 %) were considered to be good candidates and successfully received their LVADs. From epidemiologic data, we know that the number of elderly patients with terminal heart failure is much larger so one must assume that only a very small and select sample of this population is being referred. We have no way to evaluate why physicians do not refer some patients, but we can say that on three occasions, patients were self-referred from hospice and successfully implanted, implying that many patients who are acceptable candidates are not referred.

3.5   Limitations

The main limitation of this study is that observations were based on small numbers of patients from a single center participating in a multicenter clinical trial. The review of patients referred for terminal heart failure evaluation was retrospective and therefore the numbers are less reliable for total patients referred and identifying the precise reasons for refusal.

3.6   Conclusions

Advanced heart failure patients receiving HMII LVAD older than 70 years of age had similar outcomes to patients younger than 70 years of age. Older patients had acceptable length of hospital stays, adverse events, and functional recovery. Advanced age should not be used as an independent contraindication when selecting a patient for LVAD therapy. As this technology continues to improve, increasing numbers of older patients will seek centers for destination therapy. Analysis of the referral data suggests that more patients should be referred for LVAD evaluation at an experienced center, since good outcomes can be achieved in this patient cohort.

References

1. Rose EA, Gelijns AC, Moskowitz AJ, et al. Long-term mechanical left ventricular assistance for end-stage heart failure. N Engl J Med. 2001;345:1435–43.
2. El-Banayosy A, Arusoglu L, Kizner L, et al. Predictors of survival in patients bridged to transplantation with the thoratec VAD device: a single-center retrospective study on more than 100 patients. J Heart Lung Transplant. 2000;19:964–8.
3. Deng MC, Loebe M, El-Banayosy A, et al. Mechanical circulatory support for advanced heart failure: effect of patient selection on outcome. Circulation. 2001;103:231–7.
4. Granfeldt H, Koul B, Wiklund L, et al. Risk factor analysis of Swedish left ventricular assist device (LVAD) patients. Ann Thorac Surg. 2003;76:1993–8. discussion 1999.
5. Dang NC, Topkara VK, Kim BT, Mercando ML, Kay J, Naka Y. Clinical outcomes in patients with chronic congestive heart failure who undergo left ventricular assist device implantation. J Thorac Cardiovasc Surg. 2005;130:1302–9.
6. Holman WL, Kormos RL, Naftel DC, et al. Predictors of death and transplant in patients with a mechanical circulatory support device: a multi-institutional study. J Heart Lung Transplant. 2009;28:44–50.
7. Huang R, Deng M, Rogers JG, et al. Effect of age on outcomes after left ventricular assist device placement. Transplant Proc. 2006;38:1496–8.

8. Kirklin JK, Naftel DC, Kormos RL, et al. Second INTERMACS annual report: more than 1,000 primary left ventricular assist device implants. J Heart Lung Transplant. 2010;29:1–10.

9. Klotz S, Vahlhaus C, Riehl C, Reitz C, Sindermann JR, Scheld HH. Pre-operative prediction of post-VAD implant mortality using easily accessible clinical parameters. J Heart Lung Transplant. 2010;29:45–52.

10. Lietz K, Long JW, Kfoury AG, et al. Impact of center volume on outcomes of left ventricular assist device implantation as destination therapy: analysis of the Thoratec HeartMate Registry, 1998 to 2005. Circ Heart Fail. 2009;2:3–10.

11. Rao V, Oz MC, Flannery MA, Catanese KA, Argenziano M, Naka Y. Revised screening scale to predict survival after insertion of a left ventricular assist device. J Thorac Cardiovasc Surg. 2003;125:855–62.

12. Sandner SE, Zimpfer D, Zrunek P, et al. Age and outcome after continuous-flow left ventricular assist device implantation as bridge to transplantation. J Heart Lung Transplant. 2009;28:367–72.

13. Schaffer JM, Allen JG, Weiss ES, et al. Evaluation of risk indices in continuous-flow left ventricular assist device patients. Ann Thorac Surg. 2009;88:1889–96.

14. Schenk S, McCarthy PM, Blackstone EH, et al. Duration of inotropic support after left ventricular assist device implantation: risk factors and impact on outcome. J Thorac Cardiovasc Surg. 2006;131:447–54.

15. Stepanenko A, Potapov EV, Jurmann B, et al. Outcomes of elective versus emergent permanent mechanical circulatory support in the elderly: a single-center experience. J Heart Lung Transplant. 2010;29:61–5.

16. Topkara VK, Dang NC, Martens TP, et al. Bridging to transplantation with left ventricular assist devices: outcomes in patients aged 60 years and older. J Thorac Cardiovasc Surg. 2005;130:881–2.

17. Zahr F, Ootaki Y, Starling RC, et al. Preoperative risk factors for mortality after biventricular assist device implantation. J Card Fail. 2008;14:844–9.

18. Miller LW, Pagani FD, Russell SD, et al. Use of a continuous-flow device in patients awaiting heart transplantation. N Engl J Med. 2007;357:885–96.

19. Pagani FD, Miller LW, Russell SD, et al. Extended mechanical circulatory support with a continuous-flow rotary left ventricular assist device. J Am Coll Cardiol. 2009;54:312–21.

20. Slaughter MS, Rogers JG, Milano CA, et al. Advanced heart failure treated with continuous-flow left ventricular assist device. N Engl J Med. 2009;361:2241–51.

21. Rogers JG, Aaronson KD, Boyle AJ, et al. Continuous flow left ventricular assist device improves functional capacity and quality of life of advanced heart failure patients. J Am Coll Cardiol. 55:1826–34.

22. Lloyd-Jones D, Adams R, Carnethon M, et al. Heart disease and stroke statistics–2009 update: a report from the American Heart Association Statistics Committee and Stroke Statistics Subcommittee. Circulation. 2009;119:e21–181.

23. CMS. Centers for medicare and medicaid services. CMS Manual System, Pub 100–03 Medicare Coverage National Determinations, 2007. www.cms.hhs.gov. Accessed 23 July 2009.

24. CMS. Centers for medicare and medicaid services. Medicare Approved Facilities/VAD/list. http://www.cms.hhs.gov/MedicareApprovedFacilitie/VAD/list.asp. Accessed 23 July 2009.

25. Badiwala MV, Rao V. Left ventricular device as destination therapy: are we there yet? Curr Opin Cardiol. 2009;24:184–9.

26. Butler J, Geisberg C, Howser R, et al. Relationship between renal function and left ventricular assist device use. Ann Thorac Surg. 2006;81:1745–51.

27. Ma L, Fujino Y, Matsumiya G, Sawa Y, Mashimo T. Renal function with left ventricular assist devices: the poorer the preoperative renal function, the longer the recovery. Med Sci Monit. 2008;14:CR621–7.

28. Sandner SE, Zimpfer D, Zrunek P, et al. Renal function and outcome after continuous flow left ventricular assist device implantation. Ann Thorac Surg. 2009;87:1072–8.

29. Holdy K, Dembitsky W, Eaton LL, et al. Nutrition assessment and management of left ventricular assist device patients. J Heart Lung Transplant. 2005;24:1690–6.
30. Lietz K, Long JW, Kfoury AG, et al. Outcomes of left ventricular assist device implantation as destination therapy in the post-REMATCH era: implications for patient selection. Circulation. 2007;116:497–505.
31. Slaughter MS, Pagani FD, Rogers JG, et al. Clinical management of continuous-flow left ventricular assist devices in advanced heart failure. J Heart Lung Transplant. 2010;29(4 Suppl): S1–39.

Chapter 4
The Economics of Long-Term Ventricular Assist Device Therapy for Patients with End-Stage Heart Failure

Robin R. Bostic

Abstract The cost of medical and surgical treatment of advanced heart failure is significant, with surgical therapy having a higher initial cost. Medical therapy alone is expensive with nearly 50 % of expenditures in the last 6 months of life. However, surgical treatments such as heart transplantation and use of ventricular assist devices (VAD) are associated with significantly better average quality of life and functional capacity. Overall two-thirds of the estimated 50 billion dollars Medicare spends annually for the care of heart failure patients is for inpatient care. Less than 0.2 % of that total was due to cost of VADs for destination therapy (DT), mechanical circulatory support for life.

All treatment options for heart failure patients come at a significant cost. As mechanical support widens its utilization, it is important to further study and weigh the cost benefit in terms of survival, functional capacity, and quality of life improvement, as well as its relative cost compared to other heart failure treatments.

Keywords Cost • Destination therapy • Medical management

4.1 Introduction

Congestive heart failure has become a worldwide epidemic with current estimates of 5–7 million patients in the USA and 25 million patients worldwide [1]. Japan has a population of 127 million, of which 28 million are over the age of 65. It is estimated that 25 % of the population will be 65 or older by 2020. Current estimates indicate that 1–2 million people have chronic heart failure and nearly 170,000 die due to heart diseases each year [2]. In 2009, only four heart transplants were

R.R. Bostic (✉)
Thoratec Corporation, 6101 Stoneridge Drive, Pleasanton, CA 94588, USA
e-mail: Robin.bostic@thoratec.com

S. Kyo (ed.), *Ventricular Assist Devices in Advanced-Stage Heart Failure,*
DOI 10.1007/978-4-431-54466-1_4, © Springer Japan 2014

performed and only 69 between 1998 and June 2010. Two-thirds of patients on the transplant list have been waiting more than 2 years for a heart transplant with nearly 15 % waiting more than 5 years [3].

While progress has been made with current pharmacologic therapy for heart failure, an increasing number of patients become refractory to all current medical therapy and develop advanced, symptomatic heart failure. Several factors influence the prevalence of heart failure with advancing age being the most significant. It is estimated that at least 10 % of the population over 65 years of age will develop heart failure, and this age group alone is projected to double to over 70 million in the USA alone by the year 2020. Thus, the number of patients with advanced systolic heart failure will increase significantly over the next several decades [4].

While progress has been made on the management of heart failure, unfortunately the overall mortality remains very high at 5 years from diagnosis which is now estimated to be over 60 % [4, 5] may be as high as 80 % at 1 year in the most advanced stage [6]. In addition, the quality of life and functional limitations in patients with advanced heart failure are typically severe as well. The actual percentages of patients with the advanced phase of heart failure (American Heart Association Stage D) have been variably estimated to be as many as 100–150,000 of the 3.5 million people with systolic heart failure [4, 5]. These patients often require hospitalization for management of volume overload [7, 8]. In fact, heart failure has become the number one volume diagnosis (number of hospital days times number of hospital admissions in the Medicare health system), with more hospital days spent for management of heart failure than any other diagnosis. Medicare spends more than five billion each year making congestive heart failure one of the most costly episodes of care [7, 9]. Currently over two-thirds of all Medicare expenditures for the care of patients with heart failure are for inpatient services. In addition, it is clear that current medical therapy remains largely palliative, as heart failure is also the number one readmission diagnosis in the Medicare system with an estimated 20 % of patients readmitted within 30 days of hospital discharge for heart failure and over 50 % readmitted within 6 months. The prognosis of patients once they have been admitted for heart failure is also markedly reduced with a mortality as high as 10 % at 30 days and 33 % at 1 year [6, 10, 11]. These data confirm heart failure is, and will continue to be, a major healthcare issue of the future. New and more effective interventions are needed to reduce the cycle of recurrent hospitalization and improve the very poor quality of life for these patients.

4.2 Cost

4.2.1 Medical Therapy

Despite the large and increasing economic impact of heart failure, there is a paucity of data measuring the overall cost of HF care [7]. However, it is apparent that once

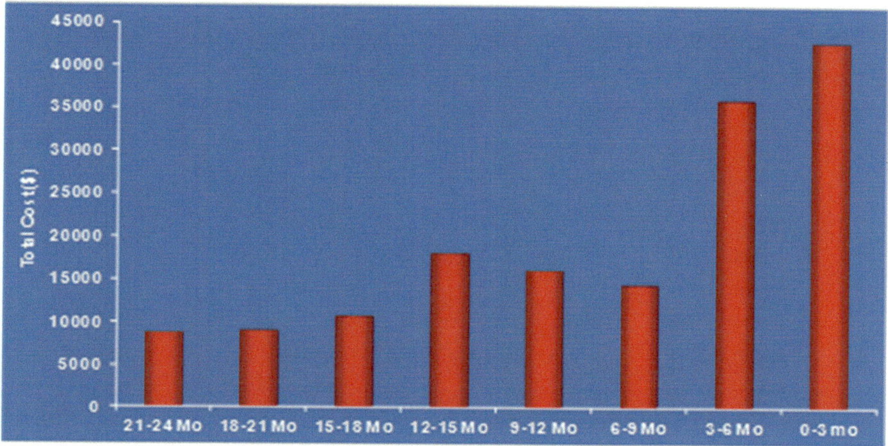

Fig. 4.1 Cost of medical therapy for end-stage heart failure patients during last 2 years of life by 3 month time periods as a percentage of the total cost

patients have reached the most advanced phase of heart failure, their prognosis worsens significantly, and the cost investment and economic impact go up substantially, yet quality of life and functional capacity typically decline [11]. Russo et al. analyzed the mean cost for the care of 52 heart failure patients during their last 2 years of life. The data was derived from the REMATCH study [6] which randomized patients with end-stage HF to either a left ventricular assist device (LVAD) or optimal medical therapy. The study analyzed data from the 52 of the 68 patients in the medical therapy arm who were Medicare beneficiaries from the time of their death, retrospectively for the 2 years prior, including all inpatient and outpatients services. The mean cost of care of these patients for the last 2 years of their life was over $160,000 per patient, with 45 % of that total, median of $83,000, spent during the last six months of life (Fig. 4.1). A good deal of the care and cost in the last 6 months was hospital based, including time in an intensive care unit, suggesting that when patients reach the most advanced phase of HF, they have a terminal prognosis and medical therapy alone has been a relatively ineffective and expensive form of therapy. Importantly, these patients were enrolled between 1998 and 2000, which was prior to the demonstration of the survival benefit and increased use and cost of internal cardio-defibrillators and biventricular pacing. When compared to other chronic conditions such as chronic obstructive lung disease and lung and pancreatic cancer, HF care in the last 6 months was 2 to 3 times greater than for the other diseases, $83,000 versus $30,000 for the other chronic illnesses [11].

LVAD Cost Effectiveness tracks with HT in trending downward over time

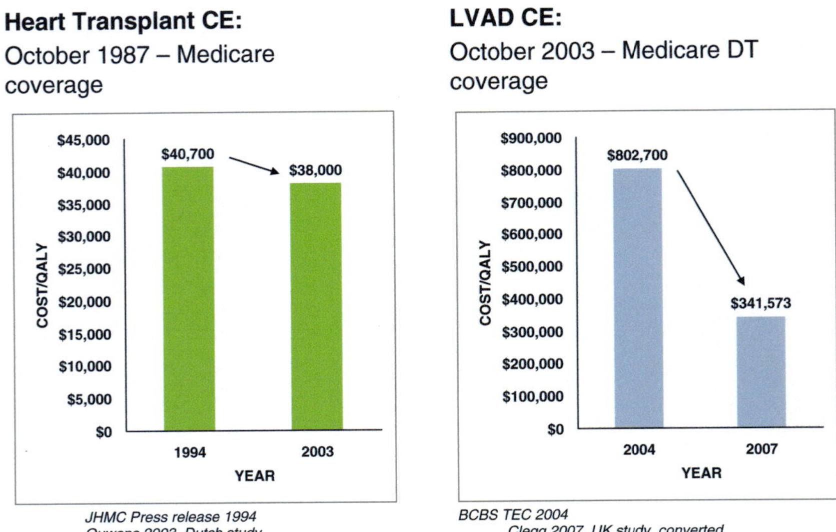

Fig. 4.2 Reduction in cost of heart transplantation over 4 year time period 1991–1995 versus reduction in cost of LVAD therapy from 1991 to 1994

4.2.2 *Surgical Therapy*

The cost of surgical therapy is also expensive but associated with trends showing a reduction in cost with increased experience. Heart transplantation is a standard form of surgical treatment of end-stage heart failure. In Japan only 169 patients were placed on the 2010 heart transplant list. In 2009, only four heart transplants were performed and only 69 between 1998 and June 2010. Two-thirds of patients on the transplant list have been waiting more than 2 years for a heart transplant with nearly 15 % waiting more than 5 years [3].

At Columbia University Medical Center, the overall average cost of heart transplant with 120 days follow-up was reported as $150,000. Despite its expense, the societal cost of heart transplant will never be prohibitively high simply because the volume of transplantations is primarily determined by the limited availability of donor hearts [12].

Increasing experience with this procedure and advances in immunosuppression were associated with 45 % reduction in cost reported for heart transplantation of nearly 45 % between 1991 and 1995, shortly after Center for Medicare/Medicaid Services (CMS) began to approve heart transplantation. Similarly a 40 % reduction in mechanical support cost was reported over a 3 year experience period between 2001 and 2004 (Fig. 4.2) after this therapy received CMS approval [13].

Table 4.1 Japanese reimbursement for VADs

Functional category: VAD set	Functional code				Fee $US (¥yen)
(1) Extracorporeal	B002	129	01		~$38,900 (¥3,130,000)
(2) Implantable (pulsatile)	B002	129	02		~$172,600 (¥13,900,000)
(3) Implantable (non-pulsatile)					
1. Magnetic levitation type	B002	129	03	01	~$224,800 (¥18,100,000)
2. Water circulation type	B002	129	03	02	~$224,800 (¥18,100,000)
(4) Water circulation circuit set	B002	129	04		~$13,000 (¥1,050,000)

Table 4.2 Impact of VAD adverse event on cost

Adverse event	Incremental costs
Impact of adverse event on cost	
No complications	$147,722
Late bleeding (after 24 h)	$52,537
Respiratory failure	$38,076
Perioperative bleeding	$21,502
Infection (other than sepsis and pump housing infection)	$37,721

The presence of postoperative bleeding, respiratory failure, and infection represents incremental hospitalization cost

Use of mechanical circulatory assist devices have become an increasing surgical treatment option for patients who deteriorate while awaiting heart transplant as well as an alternative to transplant. The cost of the index hospitalization for the patients who were randomized to LVAD therapy in the REMATCH study averaged $210,000, with a large standard deviation of $193,000 and a median cost of $145,000 (range $76,000–$733,000). The cost was approximately $100,000 for those who survived the index hospitalization and as high as $700,000 for those who had an extended intensive care unit period and did not survive hospitalization, which emphasizes the importance of patient selection in use of this therapy [14].

A more recent comparison of the cost of mechanical support for patients receiving a LVAD between 2003 and 2004 compared to patients implanted in the year 2000 showed that the length of stay had been reduced by over 25%, and the index hospitalization costs were reduced by approximately 40 % to an average of $128,000 [13]. This was in part due to a 40 % reduction in length of stay and a 44 % reduction in hospital cost; this averaged $115,000 in survivors. Slaughter et al. also reported a similar 45 % reduction in cost of the index hospitalization over a 2-year period of observation, which averaged $125,000 in their recent assessment [15].

The use of ventricular assist devices for the treatment of advanced heart failure in Japan was approved in 2000 with reimbursement of $31,600 (3,160,000¥) for external pulsatile device. As of November 2012, the HeartMate II implantable continuous-flow device was approved for use in Japan with reimbursement announced April 2013 at a rate of $180,000 (18,100,000¥) [16] (Table 4.1; Japanese VAD Reimbursement Rates).

At this time, there is no Japanese LVAD cost data, but if we see a similar trend as reported in the USA, with experience, careful patient selection and improved survival, reduction of length of stay days, and readmissions, cost will go down (Table 4.2).

4.3 Cost-Effectiveness

It is important to understand the concept of a cost-effective analysis (CEA). The American College of Physicians explains how the CEA results might be considered as the "price" of the additional outcome purchased by switching from current practice to the new strategy. If the price is low enough, the new strategy is considered "cost-effective." If a strategy is dubbed "cost-effective" and the term is used as its creators intended, it means that the new strategy is a good value. Being cost-effective does not mean the strategy saves money, and just because a strategy saves money doesn't mean that it is cost-effective. The very notion of cost-effective requires a value judgment—what you think is a good price for an additional outcome, someone else may not. What is life worth? [17].

The clinical assessment of the left ventricular device technology is evolving. It has been clearly established as clinically beneficial with a favorable technology assessment from Blue Cross Blue Shield (BCBS) Technology Assessment Committee followed by positive National Coverage Determination by CMS as the treatment for end-stage heart failure patients ineligible for heart transplant also known as destination therapy (DT) [18, 19].

The overall clinical acceptance of this therapy led to an immediate review by BCBS on whether the use of the therapy was a cost-efficient treatment. These initial studies suggested LVADs were not cost-effective, with LVAD incremental cost-effectiveness ratio (ICER) "price" as high as $802,700 (BCBS TEC), which is beyond generally accepted threshold of $50,000–100,000 per quality-adjusted life year (QALY) "value" gained [20].

More recently, an assessment of patients undergoing both acute and chronic VAD support with multiple types of first-generation mechanical assist devices suggested it was a high-cost therapy that did not meet Institute of Medicine goals for cost or outcomes when costs were analyzed out to 1 year post implant. The problem with retrospective data compiled over a number of years in a field that is evolving so rapidly is that it does not reflect current practice or outcomes [21, 22].

Using a more recent dataset from the HeartMate II Destination Therapy trial that included initial hospital stay, outpatient supplies, re-hospitalizations, and Medicare payments for professional services, the cost of LVAD therapy was compared with the cost of medical therapy to treat advanced heart failure patients. Continuous-flow LVAD patients had higher quality-adjusted life years (1.87 versus 0.37), and life years (2.42 versus 0.64), as well as higher 5-year costs ($360,407 versus $62,856) for medical management. The incremental cost-effectiveness ratio of the continuous-flow LVAD was $198,184 per QALY and $167,208 per life year, which was equivalent to a relative 75 % reduction in incremental cost-effectiveness ratio from $802, 700 per QALY in 2004. [23] This recent data demonstrate LVAD therapy has not yet achieved cost-effectiveness (strictly as per definition) in the USA (<$100,000/incremental cost-effectiveness ratio), but the improvements gained in the short term are encouraging.

The primary determinants of cost-effectiveness using current methodology are total cost, survival, and quality of life. If quality of life remains stable, combinations of cost stabilize and 2-year survival improves from 58 to 70%, and then using the same cost-effective model, the HeartMate II would meet the $100,000 ICER [24] when used as destination therapy.

However, one important deficiency in using only cost in the assessment of the effectiveness of lifesaving therapies is it omits the very important parameters of change in functional capacity and life management. The improvement in functional capacity with medical therapy for advanced heart failure is modest at best. While cardiac resynchronization therapy has been adopted as an accepted treatment of patients with advanced heart failure who meet eligibility criteria, the improvement reported at 6 months on the 6-minute walk test (6-MWT) in three recent studies was only 42 m [25, 26]. In contrast, the average increase in 6-MWT following use of a new continuous-flow design LVAD was nearly 300 m. In addition, the improvement in patient-assessed quality of life in the LVAD trial at 3 and 6 months was increased nearly 90 % from baseline and higher than has been reported for any medical therapy. Cost-effective models do not completely capture such pertinent elements as the actual quality impact to patients' lives [27].

4.4   Cost Comparison

The cost of therapy for advanced chronic diseases is often high, particularly in life-saving therapies such as chemotherapy, organ transplantation, or dialysis. Cardiac transplantation has been shown to be similar in cost to kidney and liver transplantation [28] (Fig. 4.3). When compared to similar orphan drug therapies such as treatment of end-stage renal disease or HIV-associated condition, VAD therapy has been shown in fact to be associated with lower annual cost [29, 30].

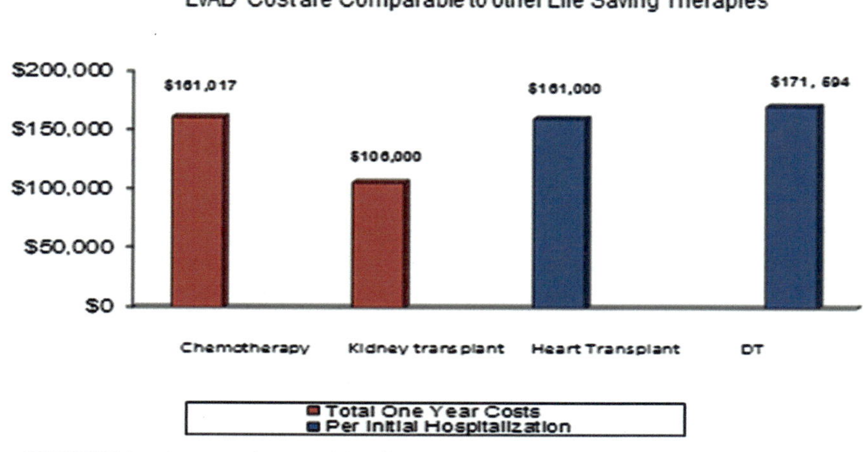

Fig. 4.3 Comparison of cost of LVAD DT therapy compared to other lifesaving therapies

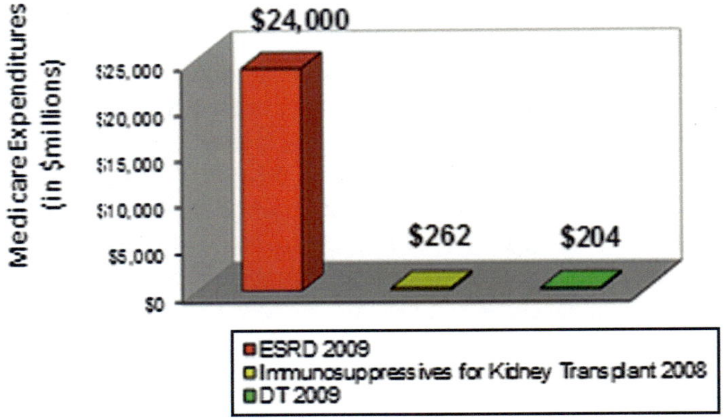

Fig. 4.4 Impact of destination therapy on Medicare budget

The annual estimated Medicare expenditures for end-stage renal disease exceed 20 billion and account for 3 % of the entire healthcare budget, whereas the use of mechanical support has estimated to total less than $204 million dollars less than 1 % [31–33] (Fig. 4.4).

4.5 Discussion

There appears to be a number of opportunities in this emerging therapy to see further cost reduction including an increased focus on the importance of patient selection [34]. Leitz et al. have demonstrated the use of a preoperative risk stratification score that can identify patients with a low likelihood of surviving the procedure and specific variables that can help influence outcome and higher likelihood of a successful outcome with mechanical support. Miller [13] verified that patient survival dramatically impacts hospital cost. Improved patient selection may have the greatest impact on survival of not only index hospitalization but also subsequent long-term survival.

Perhaps one of the most important advances that may lead to cost reduction with LVAD therapy is the development of the second generation of mechanical assist devices, which have a totally new design that utilizes continuous flow rather than pulsatile flow. The new design has allowed a reduction to one-seventh the size and one-fifth the weight compared to the first-generation device. Prospective trials of these devices have shown the complications of the new devices and hospital length of stay to be significantly lower than reported with the first-generation devices and are also associated with a significant improvement in patient-assessed quality of life and measured functional capacity [27, 35, 36]. With these more durable devices, one can project long-term implanted VADs used as support for greater than 4 years will meet the standard benchmark of $100,000 quality-adjusted life standard. Patients supported by an LVAD can return to a near-normal lifestyle, with reduced medical care costs, fewer hospitalizations, and fewer follow-up visits [15]. In addition, continued patient care is less expensive for LVAD patients than for transplant patients [37]. Higher survival rates and reduction in adverse events and length of stay for LVAD patients have also been reported by the Interagency Registry for Mechanically Assisted Circulatory Support (INTERMACs) [38] which further supports a trend of reduction in cost and improvement in cost-effectiveness. With the creation of the Japanese Mechanical Assist Circulatory System (J-MACS) Registry, data is being collected by all VAD-implanting hospitals for improving clinical assessment/management, treatment, and technologies for severe heart failure patients. This data will be beneficial for assuring patient safety in developing circulatory support devices by clarifying risks and benefits.

4.6 Conclusion

All treatment options for heart failure patients come at a significant cost. It is important as mechanical support widens in its utilization to further study and weigh the cost benefit for the various applications of LVAD therapy as well as further examine the cost of other heart failure treatments. With Medicare paying more than 39 billion dollars [1] for heart failure patients' inhospital care, it is paramount to determine at what time a VAD should be used and for what populations. The rapidly growing number of patients who become unresponsive to optimized medical therapy continues to expand rapidly and evolving therapies such as VADs need to be carefully examined as one potentially important treatment option, especially when used in patients before they reach such an advanced stage of their disease where outcomes of any therapy will be poor.

With 25 % of the Japanese population projected to be over 65 by 2020 and potentially 170,000 individuals dying from heart disease [2], it's important that lifesaving therapies such as ventricular assist devices be accessible to those patients who would most benefit, at a cost that allows health systems to provide the care.

References

1. Lloyd-Jones D, Adams RJ, Brown TM, Carnethon M, Dai S, De Simone G, Ferguson TB, Ford E, Furie K, Gillespie C, Go A, Greenlund K, Haase N, Hailpern S, Ho PM, Howard V, Kissela B, Kittner S, Lackland D, Lisabeth L, Marelli A, McDermott MM, Meigs J, Mozaffarian D, Mussolino M, Nichol G, Roger VL, Rosamond W, Sacco R, Sorlie P, Stafford R, Thom T, Wasserthiel-Smoller S, Wong ND, Wylie-Rosett J. American Heart Association Statistics Executive summary: heart disease and stroke statistics–2010 update: a report from the American Heart Association Circulation.
2. Shiba N, Shimokawa, H. Chronic heart failure in Japan: implications of the CHART studies. Vasc Health Risk Manage. 2008;4(1):103–13; 2010;121:948–54.
3. The Japan Organ Transplant Network. Organ transplanting in Japan. The Japan Organ Transplant Network. 2011. http://www.jotnw.or.jp/english/00.html. Accessed 23 June 2011.
4. Bursi F, Weston SA, Redfield MM, Jacobsen SJ, Pakhomov S, Nkomo VT, Meverden RA, Roger VL. Systolic and diastolic ventricular dysfunction in the community. JAMA. 2006;296:2209–16.
5. National Heart, Lung, and Blood Institute (NHLBI) United States. Source: National Hospital Discharge Survey (NHDS)/National Center for Health Statistics (NCHS) and National Heart, Lung, and Blood Institute; 1979–2006.
6. Rose EA, Gelinjn A, Moskowitz AD, et al. Long term mechanical left ventricular assistance for end-stage heart failure. N Eng J Med. 2001;345:1435–43.
7. Jencks S, Williams M, Coleman E. Rehospitalization among patients in the medicare fee-for-service program. N Engl J Med. 2008;360:14.
8. Loehr LR, Rosamond WD, Chang PP, Folsom AR, Chambliss LE. Heart failure incidence and survival (from the Atherosclerosis Risk in Communities Study). Am J Cardiol. 2008;101(7):1016–22.
9. Cutler DM, et al. The potential for cost savings through bundled episode payments. N Engl J Med. 2012;366:1075–7.
10. The Pharmaceuticals and Medical Device Agency, Japan. List of approved products. http://www.pmda.go.jp/english/service/list_s.html. Accessed 23 June 2011.
11. Russo MJ, Gelijns AC, Stevenson LW, et al. The cost of medical management in advanced heart failure during the final two years of life. J Card Fail. 2008;14(8):651–8.
12. DiGiorgi PL, Reel MS, Thornton B, Burton E, Naka Y, Oz MC. Heart transplant and left ventricular assist device costs. J Heart Lung Transplant. 2005;24(2):200.
13. Miller LW, Nelson KE, Bostic RR, Tong K, Slaughter MS, Long JW. Hospital costs for left ventricular assist devices for destination therapy: lower costs for implantation in the post-REMATCH era. J Heart Lung Transplant. 2006;25:778–84.
14. Oz MC, Gelijns AC, et al. Left ventricular assist devices as permanent heart failure therapy – the price of progress. Ann Surg. 2003;238:577–85.
15. Slaughter MS, Bostic R, Tong K, Russo M, Rogers JG. Temporal changes in hospital costs for left ventricular assist device implantation. J Card Surg. 2011;26:535–41.
16. Japan CHUIKYO, http://www.iryohoken.go.jp/shinryohoshu/ 2013.
17. American College of Physicians. Copyright cost effective analysis. American College of Physicians; 2012.
18. Blue Cross Blue Shield Association Technology Assessment Committee. Special report: left ventricular assist devices as destination therapy for end stage heart failure. Blue Cross Blue Shield Technol Eval Center Bull. 2004;19(2):1–29.
19. Centers for Medicare and Medicaid Services. Medicare National Coverage Determinations Manual, Chapter 1, Part 1, Section 20.9. Artificial hearts and related devices. 2003. http://www.cms.hhs.gov/manuals/103_cov_determ/ncd103c1_Part1.pdf Accessed April 2008.
20. Blue Cross Blue Shield Association Medical Advisory Panel. Special report: cost effectiveness of left ventricular assist devices as destination therapy for end stage heart failure. Blue Cross Blue Shield Technol Eval Center Bull. 2004;19(2):1–29.

21. Hernandez AF, Grab JD, Gammie JS, et al. A decade of short-term outcomes in post cardiac surgery ventricular assist device implantation: data from the Society of Thoracic Surgeons' National Cardiac Database. Circulation. 2007;116(6):606–12.
22. Hutchinson J, Scott DA, Clegg AJ, Loveman E, Royle P, Bryant J, Colquitt JL. Cost-effectiveness of left ventricular-assist devices in end-stage heart failure. Expert Rev Cardiovasc Ther. 2008;6:175–85.
23. Rogers JG, Bostic RR, Tong KB, Adamson R, Russo M, Slaughter MS. Cost-effectiveness analysis of continuous-flow left ventricular assist devices as destination therapy. Circulation. 2012;5:10–6.
24. Miller LW, Rogers JG. Cost of ventricular assist devices: can we afford the progress? Circulation. 2013;127:743–8.
25. Strickberger SA, Conti J. Daoud EG et al on behalf of the council on clinical cardiology and the heart rhythm society. Patient selection for cardiac resynchronization therapy. Circulation. 2005;111:2146–50.
26. Lindenfeld J, Fledman AM, Saxon L, et al. The effect of resynchronization therapy with or without a defibrillator on survival and hospitalizations in patients with New York Heart Association Class IV heart failure. Circulation. 2007;115:204–12.
27. Rogers JG, Aaronson KD, Boyle AJ, Russell SD, Milano CA, Pagani FD, Edwards BS, Park S, John R, Conte JV, Farrar DJ, Slaughter MS. Continuous flow left ventricular assist device improves functional capacity and quality of life of advanced heart failure patients. J Am Coll Cardiol. 2010;55:1826–34.
28. Oostenbrink JG, et al. Transpl Int. 2006;18(4):437–43.
29. Vupputuri S. Epidemiology and costs of chronic kidney disease in North Carolina. N C Med J. 2008;69(3):205–7.
30. Foley RN, Collins AJ. Cost of ESRD to medicare. J Am Soc Nephrol. 2007:2644–8.
31. CMS. Medicare/medicaid budget. 2010. http://www.hhs.gov/about/FY2012budget/cmsfy12cj_revised.pdf.
32. Knauf F, Aronson PS. Cost of ESRD. J Am Soc Nephrol. 2009;20(10):2093–7.
33. CMS MEDPAR. MS-DRG1 annual costs of medicare DT patients. 2010.
34. Lietz K, Long JW, Kfoury AG, Slaughter MS, Silver MA, Milano CA, Rogers JG, Naka Y, Mancini D, Miller LW. Outcomes of left ventricular assist device implantation as destination therapy in the post-REMATCH era: implications for patient selection. Circulation. 2007;116:497–505.
35. Miller LW, Pagani FD, Russell SD, John R, Boyle AJ, Aaronson KD, Conte JV, Naka Y, Mancini D, Delgado RM, Macgillivray TE, Farrar DJ, Frazier OH. Use of a continuous-flow device in patients awaiting heart transplantation. N Engl J Med. 2007;357:885–96.
36. Slaughter MS, Rogers JG, Milano CA, Russell SD, Conte JV, Feldman D, Sun B, Tatooles AJ, Delgado III RM, Long JW, Wozniak TC, Ghumman W, Farrar DJ, Frazier OH. Advanced heart failure treated with continuous-flow left ventricular assist device. N Engl J Med. 2009;361:2241–51.
37. Goldstein D, Sileo A, Baker L, Vandevoort K, Cotter P. Contemporary continuous flow devices: how much does it cost to keep a patient on support for one year? J Heart Lung Transplant. 2012;30:S85.
38. Kirklin JK, Naftel DC, Kormos RL, Stevenson LW, Pagani FD, Miller MA, Baldwin JT, Young JB. The fourth INTERMACS annual report: 4,000 implants and counting. J Heart Lung Transplant. 2012;31:117–26.

Chapter 5
Improving Clinical Outcomes:
A Targeted Approach

Mark Jay Zucker and Hassan Baydoun

Abstract Mechanical cardiac support, in the form of an implantable left ventricular assist device, is no longer considered an experimental intervention for patients with advanced left ventricular dysfunction. The considerable expense associated with each implant, however, makes it incumbent upon the clinician to ensure that only appropriate and timely referred candidates are selected. Medical and psychosocial considerations are paramount and both have been repeatedly shown to impact long-term outcomes. Patients with limited support systems, multiple comorbidities, marginal hemodynamics, right heart dysfunction, frailty, and hematologic problems such as hypercoagulability and/or coagulopathy may not be ideal device recipients. Predictive algorithms have been developed to help identify high- and low-risk patients, but the algorithms often prove inaccurate. Regardless of the estimated risk, all efforts must be made preoperatively to reduce or even eliminate any potential medical problems that might increase the surgical risk. Intraoperative management is, of course, critical as well. Beta-agonists, inotropes, and short-acting pulmonary vasodilators such as nitric oxide or inhaled prostacyclin should be introduced in the operating room, as needed. Successful separation from cardiopulmonary bypass inevitably requires patience and careful monitoring of right ventricular size, shape, and function either via direct vision or with transesophageal echocardiography. Postoperative challenges to be anticipated include gastrointestinal bleeding secondary to arteriovenous malformations, pump thrombosis, ischemic and hemorrhagic cerebrovascular events, and aortic insufficiency. The possibility of infection must be entertained at all times. Standard prophylactic antibiotic regimens should be set

M.J. Zucker (✉)
Newark Beth Israel Medical Center, New Jersey Medical School, Rutgers University,
201 Lyons Avenue, Newark, NJ 07112, USA
e-mail: mzucker@barnabashealth.org

H. Baydoun
Department of Internal Medicine, Staten Island University Hospital, Staten Island, NY 10305, USA

S. Kyo (ed.), *Ventricular Assist Devices in Advanced-Stage Heart Failure,*
DOI 10.1007/978-4-431-54466-1_5, © Springer Japan 2014

in place at all implanting centers based upon institution-specific data. These considerations in association with early ambulation and aggressive rehabilitation should help ensure a successful long-term outcome.

Keywords Aortic insufficiency • Complications • Long-term outcomes • Mechanical cardiac support • Patient selection • Right heart failure • Risk algorithms • Ventricular assist device

5.1 Introduction

Although more than 2,300 donor hearts were procured in the United States in 2012 [1], it is understood that thousands of other individuals might also have benefitted from transplantation had a donor heart been found [2]. Unfortunately, despite public education and the work of the organ procurement organizations, the number of acceptable donor hearts is unlikely to increase sufficiently at any time in the near future to accommodate this unmet need. For these individuals, or for those individuals listed for transplantation who become hemodynamically unstable prior to the identification of a suitable donor heart, the only realistic option might be mechanical circulatory support.

Early attempts at mechanical cardiac support by Dennis in 1961 [3] and Spencer in 1963 [4] relied upon extracorporeal roller pumps with inflow and outflow connections between the left atrium and ascending aorta or between the left ventricle and femoral artery, respectively. Pneumatically actuated pulsatile devices were not introduced until the mid-1970s [5, 6]. Most of these devices were extracorporeal as well, although Cooley and Norman did conduct a trial with the TECO Model VII intra-abdominal left ventricular assist device (ALVAD) in the mid- to late 1970s [6]. More recent efforts at mechanical circulatory support in the United States have relied upon both paracorporeal and implantable left ventricular assist systems marketed by an ever increasing number of device manufacturers.

The first commercially approved pulsatile ventricular assist system intended for hemodynamic and circulatory support in patients with cardiogenic shock was the HeartMate XVE. The device, which is no longer in production, was the first left ventricular assist device (LVAD) to be studied for "destination" therapy (DT). The REMATCH trial, as the study was known, is now considered a landmark endeavor [7]. For the first time, mechanical support was shown to be more effective than optimal medical management. One-year survival in patients randomized to an LVAD was 52.1 % as compared to 24.7 % for patients randomized to medical therapy ($p=0.002$). At 2 years, the relative difference was even more pronounced—22.9 % vs. 8.1 %—but statistical significance was not achieved due to sample size ($p=0.09$). Dramatic improvements were noted in the quality of life for those patients who were implanted with an LVAD. As a result of the study, in late 2002 the device's manufacturer received regulatory approval from the FDA to market the LVAD as an alternative to medical therapy for non-transplant candidates.

Many lessons were learned from the LVAD experiences of the late 1990s and early 2000s. Perhaps the most significant, however, was the importance of timing of referral and implantation—the sooner, the better. Unfortunately, familiarity with and acceptance of this technology remained (and to a large extent still remains) limited in the non-heart failure cardiology community. Patients are too often referred for LVAD placement by their cardiologist as a "bridge to transplantation" (BTT) or for "destination therapy" only as a "last resort" intervention.

5.2   Selection of Candidates

As part of the conditions of approval for many of the implantable devices the FDA mandated that demographic, clinical, and outcome data be entered into a registry for each patient implanted with a commercially approved device. As a result, the Interagency Registry for Mechanically Assisted Circulatory Support (INTERMACS) was established. The inclusion of the patient's data requires individual patient consent. Thus, INTERMACS is not all inclusive. Nonetheless, it has provided the mechanical support community with a considerable amount of data and has reaffirmed the observation noted above—the sooner, the better. Outcomes have been consistently worse in patients classified as INTERMACS 1 and 2 (as defined in Table 5.1) than in patients classified as INTERMACS 3–7 [8–10]. Today, it is widely acknowledged that individuals in cardiogenic shock may not be ideal candidates for urgent placement of an implantable device. Instead, these patients may be better served by temporary mechanical support devices (such as balloon pumps, transaortic axial flow pumps, paracorporeal VADs, or perhaps extracorporeal membrane oxygenation (ECMO)) to first optimize their hemodynamics, respiratory status, renal status, and acid–base balance. Stated again, timing of device placement and choice of device are both critical to ensure success [11].

Not all patients referred for VAD placement are candidates for VAD placement. Multiple contraindications, exclusions, psychosocial considerations, and technical

Table 5.1 INTERMACS patient profile

Patient profile	Patient characteristics
1	Critical cardiogenic shock despite escalating support
2	Progressive decline with inotrope dependence
3	Clinically stable with mild to moderate inotrope dependence
4	Recurrent, not refractory, advanced heart failure that can be stabilized with intervention
5	Exertion intolerant but comfortable at rest and able to perform activities of daily living with slight difficulty
6	Exertion limited; able to perform mild activity, but fatigue results within a few minutes of any meaningful physical exertion
7	Advanced NYHA functional class III

challenges can derail the best of intentions. Each patient must be individually evaluated. Family support systems must be assessed by an appropriate social worker or VAD coordinator. The importance of a reliable "companion" cannot be overstated. General guidelines and recommendations set forth in the literature must be considered [12]. Not unexpectedly, national and international organizations have all published recommendations and guidelines for the use of mechanical cardiac support including the Heart Failure Society of America, the European Society of Cardiology, and the AHA/ACC [13–16]. The recent recommendations published in Circulation in November 2012 [17] are representative and are summarized below.

For the BTT population, mechanical cardiac support is indicated in patients who have failed optimal medical management and are at risk for death before a donor heart is identified (Class I/Level of Evidence (LOE) B). Exclusion criteria when used as a bridge to transplantation are relatively few simply because the patient's appropriateness for a VAD can usually be assumed based upon the fact that the patient has been deemed an acceptable candidate for transplantation. Most of the exclusions are related to technical challenges or the presence of biventricular failure. These include:

1. Body surface area <1.5 m^2
2. Age >70–72
3. Hemodialysis-dependent renal failure
4. Severe right ventricular dysfunction
5. Intractable ventricular tachycardia
6. Active systemic infection
7. Severe hypercoagulability
8. Prolonged acute kidney injury
9. Recent CPR resulting in significant renal dysfunction or respiratory failure

In contrast to BTT, the indications for (and timing of) VAD placement for DT are less clear-cut, and the field continues to evolve. The Circulation publication addressed this subject as well. DT is indicated for the treatment of patients with:

1. Advanced heart failure—regardless of the need for inotropes (Class IIa/LOE B)
2. Advanced heart failure in patients failing optimal medical management (Class I/ LOE B)
3. Advanced heart failure and pulmonary hypertension rendering them ineligible for transplantation (Class IIa/LOE B)
4. Advanced heart failure and obesity rendering them ineligible for transplantation (Class IIb/LOE B)

Notably absent from the list set forth above is the issue of age. In contrast to transplantation where age is a serious consideration, age is less of a concern in the world of mechanical cardiac support. In fact, most programs will entertain LVAD placement in individuals up to the age of 80 years, if not older, assuming that they are otherwise acceptable candidates with no other life-threatening comorbidities.

5.3 Determinants of Risk

5.3.1 Risk Algorithms for Perioperative Morbidity and Mortality

Multiple different models have been developed to predict operative risk. The value of these models was recently reviewed by the United States Veterans Administration Quality Enhancement Research Initiative's (QUERI) Evidence-based Synthesis Program (ESP) [18]. None of these models was felt to be truly reliable. Nevertheless, there are some commonalities that seem to cross all of the models. As such, some of the predictive models are listed in abridged form below. Note that these models address global risk and are not specifically addressing the risk of right heart failure which is discussed separately later in this chapter.

One of the earliest risk models (using HeartMate VE data) was presented in the mid-1990s by Dr. Mehmet Oz [19] and suggested that the outcome was worse if:

1. The urine output is <30 cc/h.
2. The CVP is >16 mmHg.
3. The PT is >16 s.
4. The patient has previously undergone a median sternotomy.
5. The patient is on a ventilator.
6. The platelet count has recently fallen.
7. The fibrinogen is <300.

Over the years, the risk scoring algorithm was modified by Rao [20] with some points being added and some being removed. For a point score >5, the perioperative mortality was 46 %, whereas if the point score was ≤5, the perioperative mortality was only 12 % ($p<0.001$).

1. Ventilator dependent	4 points
2. Prior median sternotomy	2 points
3. Previous LVAD	2 points
4. CVP >16 mmHg	1 point
5. PT >16 s	1 point

Historically, the most widely used score had been the Leitz–Miller score derived from a cohort of 222 HeartMate XVE recipients, all of whom were included in the Thoratec DT registry [21]. Nine preoperative risk factors were identified which predicted 90-day mortality and 1-year survival:

1. Platelets <148,000	7 points
2. Albumin <3.3 g/dL	5 points
3. INR >1.1	4 points
4. Vasodilator therapy	4 points
5. Mean PAP <25 mmHg	3 points
6. AST >45	2 points
7. Hematocrit <34 %	2 points
8. BUN >51 mg/dL	2 points
9. Lack of IV inotropic support	2 points

Low-risk patients were those whose point total was ≤16 (69 % 1-year survival), whereas high-risk patients were those whose point total was >16 (13 % 1-year survival).

In 2009, the Hopkins group reported in the Annals of Thoracic Surgery a comparison of five risk scoring algorithms [22], three of which are described above. The last two are not LVAD-specific risk assessment algorithms whatsoever—the APACHE II score[1] and the Seattle Heart Failure Model.[2] Surprisingly, the best predictor of postoperative outcome was the SHFM.

In 2013, Cowgers proposed an updated HeartMate II Risk Score based upon an analysis of 1,122 patients enrolled in the HeartMate II BTT and DT trials between the years 2005 and 2010 [23]. This was the first large-scale analysis evaluating risk factors in patients with axial flow rather than pulsatile-flow devices. Only five variables (based upon multivariable analysis) were shown to be predictive of outcome—older age, hypoalbuminemia, renal dysfunction, coagulopathy, and implantation at a less experienced center.

5.3.2 Assessment of Right Heart Function

One of the most important challenges to face the transplant physician and surgeon regardless of whether the LVAD is being implanted for a "bridge" or "destination" indication is right heart failure. As the number and variety of LVADs increases, this issue will become increasingly problematic. In theory, one would anticipate that this problem would occur more frequently in non-ischemic cardiomyopathy patients with biventricular dysfunction than in ischemic patients with primarily left-sided dysfunction. To date, no tested/validated algorithms capable of consistently predicting the likelihood of RV dysfunction exist. Nonetheless, some algorithms have been proposed including an RV failure score published in early 2008 by Aaronson based upon an analysis of 197 implants performed at the University of Michigan, 68 of

---

[1] The APACHE II score was developed from a multi-institutional cohort of 5,815 critically ill patients and consists of 13 preoperative variables: temperature, mean arterial pressure, heart rate, respiratory rate, partial pressure of arterial oxygen or alveolar–arterial oxygen gradient if the fraction of inspired oxygen is 50 % or more, arterial pH, serum sodium, serum potassium, serum creatinine, hematocrit, white blood cell count, Glasgow Coma Score, and age. See Crit Care Med. 1985;13:818–29.

[2] SHFM was derived from a cohort of 1,125 New York Heart Association (NYHA) class IIIB or IV patients. It uses 21 variables weighted by hazard ratio: age, gender, NYHA class, weight, ejection fraction, systolic blood pressure, presence of ischemic cardiomyopathy, daily furosemide equivalent dose, inotrope use, statin use, allopurinol use, angiotensin-converting enzyme use, β-blocker use, angiotensin receptor blocker use, potassium-sparing diuretic use, implantable cardioverter-defibrillator use, hemoglobin, lymphocyte percent on complete blood count differential, serum uric acid, serum cholesterol, and serum sodium. For the purposes of the Hopkins analysis, two additional variables were added: intra-aortic balloon pump or ventilator or both and inotrope therapy. See Circulation. 2006;113:1424–33.

which were complicated by RV failure [24]. In this analysis, RV failure was defined as the need for postoperative intravenous inotropic support for >14 days, inhaled nitric oxide for >48 h, the need for right-sided circulatory support, or hospital discharge on an inotrope. Predictors of right heart failure based upon a multivariable logistic regression model were defined as:

1. The need for preoperative vasopressors	4 points
2. An AST/SGOT >80	2 points
3. A bilirubin >2.0	2.5 points
4. A creatinine >2.3	3 points
RV failure score	*Hazard ratio of RV failure*
≥5.5	7.6
4.0–5	0 2.8
≤3.0	0.49

Interestingly, the RAP and transpulmonary gradient were not independent predictors of RV failure in this study. At present, this algorithm is not widely used.

A number of other analyses, also published between 2008 and 2010, focused on similar variables [25, 26]. Unfortunately, none of these risk prediction models/scores has achieved widespread acceptance probably because their predictive accuracy remains only fair, at best. The additional models are summarized below:

Fitzpatrick (risk increases with score >50)	Cardiac index <2.2	18
	RVSWI <0.25	18
	Severe RV dysfunction	17
	Creatinine >1.9	17
	Prior CT surgery	16
	Systolic BP <96	13
Kirklin (INTERMACS 2nd report)	Intubation	
	Hypotension	
	Vasopressors	
	Abnormal AST	
	Increased bilirubin	
	Increased creatinine	
	Decreased RVSWI	
	Increased CVP/PCW	

In 2010, Kormos reviewed the outcomes of 484 patients implanted with a HeartMate II during the BTT trial [27]. Right ventricular failure was defined as the need for a right ventricular assist device (RVAD), the need for inotropic support for 14 or more days after implantation, and/or the need for inotropic support starting more than 14 days after implantation. Six percent of patients needed an RVAD, 7 % of patients needed nitric oxide, and 7 % of patients required late inotropic support. Multivariate analysis revealed that each of the following three variables predicted a poor outcome, with the least predictive being renal dysfunction.

Ventilator support
CVP/PCWP >0.63
BUN >39

A recent study done by Korabathina evaluated a newer hemodynamic index—the pulmonary artery pulsatility index (PaPi). Although PaPi is intended to identify patients with inferior wall myocardial infarctions at risk of developing right ventricular dysfunction it may have a role in the world of LVADs. The index is calculated as the pulmonary artery pulse pressure/right atrial pressure [28, 29].

One of the most recently described approaches to predicting risk of RV failure after LVAD implantation is to measure RV free wall peak longitudinal strain [30] or RV global longitudinal myocardial strain using velocity vector imaging [31, 32]. This is a new technique that may eventually become more widely used as the software becomes more widely available.

5.3.3 Frailty Considerations

Preoperative hemodynamic, hepatic, and renal parameters do not always tell the whole story. Even with fairly acceptable parameters, some patients are still just too debilitated or "frail" to tolerate the stresses associated with implantation of an LVAD. How to identify those patients has been problematic. A similar problem faced the designers of the Medtronic CoreValve™ study in which the degree of frailty needed to be calculated to help define surgical risk [33, 34]. Ultimately, the CoreValve™ investigators adopted a frailty index to help quantitate that which is sometimes intangible. The frailty index was not intended to actually define who would or would not do well. It simply proposed some additional criteria to evaluate when considering a patient's candidacy for a major operation such as an aortic valve replacement and may be applicable in one way or another to LVAD placement as well, although this has yet to be studied or proven. Nevertheless, frailty may be an important predictor of outcome postimplantation [35].

5.3.4 Miscellaneous

In addition to the various hemodynamic, hepatic, hematologic, and renal parameters touched upon above, a multitude of concurrent cardiac problems other than right heart failure can also complicate the preoperative situation. These include mitral, tricuspid, and aortic valve disease, coronary artery disease, and intracardiac shunts. All of these problems need to be recognized and potentially addressed at the time of device placement.

5.4 Optimizing Preoperative and Intraoperative Parameters

Understanding the variables associated with surgical morbidity and mortality allows the clinician to address and potentially reduce or eliminate the risk factor prior to surgery and hopefully improve the outcome. Some variables are easier to address than others. An elevated INR due to chronic anticoagulation therapy, for example, can be easily reversed. Other variables such as ventilator-dependent respiratory failure are more difficult to manage.

5.4.1 Hematologic Parameters

If at all possible, patients should not be taken to the operating room for device implantation with an elevated INR secondary to chronic warfarin therapy. Ideally, warfarin should be stopped for a sufficient period of time to permit the INR to normalize [11]. If anticoagulation is needed due to an underlying medical problem, the patient should be converted as soon as practical to an intravenous agent such as unfractionated heparin or in the presence of heparin-induced thrombocytopenia to a direct thrombin inhibitor. In those instances where device placement must be performed urgently, the use of preoperative vitamin K and fresh frozen plasma (FFP) must be considered. Even so, the risk of bleeding is significant. Intraoperative and postoperative FFP, cryoprecipitate, and platelets are likely to be needed. The safety and efficacy of recombinant factor VIIa in this situation has not been established [36].

Many of the LVAD recipients are undergoing device placement as treatment for chronic end-stage ischemic heart disease. As such, the probability is high that the patient will be on an antiplatelet agent such as aspirin, clopidogrel, or perhaps one of the newer agents such as prasugrel, rivaroxaban, or apixaban. As with warfarin, stopping the agents would be ideal. Realistically, however, this is not always advisable. Measuring platelet function by thromboelastography might provide some information as to the degree of platelet dysfunction but from a practical point of view will not change the plan. Adequate platelets, preferably single donor, should be available.

One hematologic issue that needs to be recognized and addressed prior to device implantation yet is often overlooked is the presence of a hypercoagulable state [37]. The most common cause is probably heparin-induced thrombocytopenia, but other causes such as anticardiolipin antibody syndrome, factor V Leiden mutation, proteins S and C deficiency, methylenetetrahydrofolate reductase mutation, and prothrombin 20210 gene mutation are not infrequently seen. Each of these antibodies, deficiencies, and/or mutations can increase the risk of thrombosis, not an insignificant concern in the presence of a mechanical device. Referral to a hematologist for specific treatment recommendations is appropriate [38].

5.4.2 Right Heart Function

Reducing the risk of right heart dysfunction is critical to ensuring a positive clinical outcome [39]. INTERMACS data clearly demonstrates more serious events and worse outcomes in patients requiring biventricular support [40, 41]. Multiple preoperative and intraoperative tricks and techniques have been proposed, some based on randomized trials and others based solely upon expert opinion and anecdotes

[27, 42–48]. Almost all experts agree that the explanation for RV dysfunction is multifactorial and includes intrinsic contractility issues, geometric issues related to septal interdependence, and afterload. Each of these causes needs to be addressed.

Inotropic support in one form or another is commonly used during the early postoperative period [24]. Some programs prefer pure inotropes or vasodilators such as dobutamine and milrinone while others due to concerns over excess vasodilation and hypotension opt for beta-agonists such as isoproterenol in combination with epinephrine and a pressor such as dopamine or vasopressin. Anecdotal experience suggests that intravenous thyroid hormone (liothyronine) may be of some benefit in persistent right heart dysfunction [49, 50]. This has never been proven and is an off-label indication.

As noted, afterload in the form of an increased pulmonary vascular resistance may play a significant role in the development of post-LVAD RV dysfunction [51]. For this reason, hemodynamic measurements are routinely assessed in all patients being considered for LVAD implantation [52]. The presence of pulmonary hypertension, in and of itself, is generally not of significant concern. In fact, the ability to generate a systolic pulmonary pressure in excess of 35–40 mmHg may actually portend a good prognosis, especially in the presence of a low right atrial pressure. An elevated transpulmonary gradient or pulmonary vascular resistance due to long-standing heart failure or long-standing mitral regurgitation, for example, is more concerning. How to address this issue varies depending upon the etiology. In some cases inotropes and/or diuretics are needed. In other cases, preoperative pulmonary vasodilator therapy might be indicated.

Regardless of a patient's baseline RV afterload, the hemodynamic situation facing the right ventricle in the operating room during and after initiation of LVAD support is greatly altered. Blood transfusions, intravenous pressors, increased RV venous return, epicardial ventricular pacing, and changes in RV shape and septal function all create an environment favoring RV dysfunction. For this reason, many centers (although not all) introduce inhaled nitric oxide (NO) or inhaled prostaglandins prior to or shortly after initiating LVAD support [53–57]. Both interventions have been shown to lower pulmonary artery pressure and pulmonary vascular resistance (PVR). No large-scale randomized trials have been performed. In a fairly recent randomized trial, however, it was demonstrated that the use of NO at 40 ppm in the perioperative period did not achieve significance for the endpoint of reduction of RV dysfunction although it did reduce time on mechanical ventilation, length of hospital or intensive care unit stay, and the need for RVAD support after LVAD placement [53]. A third option available to address postoperative pulmonary hypertension is phosphodiesterase type 5A inhibition which has also been shown to result in a significant decrease in PVR when compared with control patients [58].

It has been suggested that the risk of early postoperative RV failure after placement of an axial flow pump can be reduced by maintaining a relatively low RPM [42, 59]. No such suggestion has yet been made for centrifugal pumps. (The flatter HQ curve seen with centrifugal devices means that LV unloading may not change as much with small changes in RPM.) In theory, at least with axial pumps, small decreases in RPM mean less unloading of the LV which should help to maintain normal RV shape by minimizing septal shift. While there may be some truth to this, the benefit of low RPMs with respect to RV function must be balanced against the need for forward flow and the risk of pump thrombosis which may be increased if one runs the pump at a slower speed.

If the patient does develop RV failure, treatment options depend upon the timing and reason for the dysfunction [46, 60, 61]. For intraoperative problems, one must rule out unexpected technical challenges and errors. These include malposition of the apical conduit, aortic insufficiency, and twisted outflow grafts, all of which may result in inadequate LV unloading and increased RV afterload. Alternatively, perhaps the problem is simply a cold or ischemic RV. It is for the former reason that most surgeons now implant LVADs during normothermia [62]. It is for the latter reason that patients undergoing LVAD placement also undergo an assessment of coronary anatomy. If indicated, the RCA may be bypassed. Other causes of increased RV afterload include an elevated baseline PVR or an acutely elevated PVR due to bleeding and the subsequent administration of blood products.

Intraoperative surgical techniques adopted by many centers to reduce the risk of RV failure include maintaining normothermia, avoiding cardioplegia, intraoperative hemoconcentration (2–4 L), ensuring a balanced intraventricular septum by TEE, and avoiding air emboli. It should be self-evident that bleeding must be minimized. Clearly, this last recommendation can be challenging. As noted previously, patients should generally not be on antiplatelet agents such as aspirin, clopidogrel, prasugrel, rivaroxaban, and apixaban or anticoagulants such as warfarin, ticagrelor, and dabigatran in the immediate preoperative period.

How one weans from cardiopulmonary bypass (CPB) is critical [63]. The RV cannot be allowed to distend. The mean systemic blood pressure should be maintained at least at 65–70 mmHg. The CVP should probably be in the range of 13–17 mmHg although each case needs to be individually evaluated. Lower CVPs are not necessarily better as they may reflect an inadequate RV preload. Higher CVPs suggest RV failure. LVAD flow should be initiated while still on CPB. RPMs (for the HeartMate II device) should start at approximately 6,500 and then be increased over the next 10–15 min as CPB is weaned off. Some centers leave the operating room with an RPM of 8,000 while others prefer to leave the operating room with a higher RPM. Almost certainly, there is no single correct recommendation. RPMs should be adjusted to the clinical situation and guided by intraoperative TEE or early postoperative ImaCor hTEE™ assessment of septal position, RV size and function, and LV size. Regardless of the initial setting, within 3–6 h of arrival in the CTICU, the RPMs should be increased to at least 8,600 to ensure that forward flow through the device is adequate.

One thing is clear—disagreement exists among highly respected CT surgeons as to whether a higher RPM is better or worse when it comes to RV function. In those instances in which RV failure does develop intraoperatively, it may be possible to avoid the need for an RVAD by providing temporary RV support by placing an arterial cannula from the CPB circuit into the PA and perfusing the pulmonary circuit for an hour or so. Weaning should then be reattempted prior to committing the patient to a hybrid-type RVAD (CentriMag™ or TandemHeart™) [64].

5.4.3   Intra-/Perioperative Anticoagulation

Heparin (or a derivative) is often administered preoperatively to minimize the risk of intraventricular thrombus formation. Regardless of whether heparin was infusing preoperatively or not, it is normally administered in fairly high dose during LVAD implantation. Once the LVAD has been successfully implanted and the flow generated by the device shown to be adequate, protamine is administered to reverse the effects of heparin. The role of postoperative heparin for the HeartMate II device is less clear and seems to be institution specific [65, 66]. Whereas in the past heparin was routinely introduced once early bleeding was brought under control, more recent guidelines recommend heparin postoperatively when low-flow conditions exist or when otherwise medically indicated [67]. As a result of the guideline modifications, many centers now proceed directly to anticoagulation with warfarin. Some centers, however, still bridge patients in the early postoperative period with heparin electing to introduce warfarin between days 3 and 5 postoperatively. Occasionally, bivalirudin or argatroban is used in lieu of heparin in patients with heparin-induced thrombocytopenia, but this is not recommended by the manufacturer [68–73]. There is no experience with the use of other novel oral anticoagulants.

Ideally, anticoagulation should not be discontinued in LVAD recipients. However, there are more than a few case reports and anecdotes describing situations in patients with HeartMate II devices in which anticoagulation was discontinued of necessity and in some cases permanently, especially after major gastrointestinal bleeding [74–76]. Most of the time, at least with respect to the HeartMate II device, few untoward effects were noted. Nevertheless, discontinuing warfarin is not recommended in the absence of a strong and compelling reason.

In those instances where oral anticoagulation must be discontinued, the risk needs to be clearly reviewed with the patient. Some data is available to help guide that discussion. Boyle, in 2013, reviewed the bleeding and thrombosis rates in 956 HM II patients, all of whom were on anticoagulation. Although the data has yet to be formally published, the analysis demonstrated that female gender increased the risk for both ischemic and hemorrhagic strokes, gastrointestinal bleeding, and pump thrombosis. Perhaps unexpectedly, age ≤ 65 years was a risk factor for hemorrhagic stroke. Diabetes was a risk factor for ischemic stroke. Boyle concluded that men >65 years might be more able to tolerate a lower INR than other patient cohorts. Naturally, this data applies only to the HM II device and further confirmation is needed [77].

It is critical to realize that not all pumps are alike and that anticoagulation protocols are not interchangeable. For example, the manufacturer of the HeartMate II recommends maintaining an INR of 2.0±0.5 [78], and the manufacturer of the HeartWare HVAD pump recommends maintaining an INR in the range of 2.0–3.0 but probably closer to 2.3–2.7. Likewise, the dose of aspirin is not necessarily identical either. HeartMate II recipients are not infrequently maintained on 81 mg per day, but HeartWare HVAD recipients may well need a slightly higher dose of 325 mg per day as there may be a higher pump thrombosis rate when lower doses of aspirin are used [76].

5.4.4   Valvular Heart Disease

Not infrequently, patients with end-stage left ventricular dysfunction present with valvular heart disease either secondary to the LV dysfunction or as a cause of the LV dysfunction. Even mild aortic insufficiency can become a serious problem over time, especially with non-pulsatile devices in which the valve often does not open and thus faces a constant pressure of 80 mmHg or greater resulting in pansystolic regurgitation. Blood ejected through the LVAD will leak backwards through the incompetent aortic valve into the left ventricle and then into the LVAD. Pump output will be excellent; however, net forward flow may be moderately to severely compromised. Placement of an aortic valve prosthesis may be required but mechanical prostheses tend to clot [79, 80]. The outcomes with bioprostheses have been marginally better. Over-sewing the aortic valve (recognizing that pump thrombosis will likely be a fatal event should it occur) has also been tried with varying success [81–83].

In contrast to aortic insufficiency, mild to no more than moderate mitral insufficiency, in the presence of an unloaded left ventricle, is generally not a problem [84]. Moderate to severe or severe mitral insufficiency may require a concurrent annuloplasty. Different institutions handle this problem differently and no consensus exists on what to do with 3+ or 4+ mitral regurgitation [85].

Tricuspid regurgitation of more than a mild degree may worsen right ventricular function and indirectly compromise left-sided filling [86]. If feasible, consideration should be given to placement of a tricuspid annuloplasty ring or suture repair as it has been shown that at least in patients with significant tricuspid regurgitation concomitant tricuspid procedures are associated with improved early clinical outcomes [87].

5.4.5   Coronary Artery Disease

For at least three reasons, simultaneous aortocoronary artery bypass grafting may be needed in selected cases. First and foremost is the possibility that unrecognized RV ischemia may contribute to intra- or early post-op RV dysfunction. For this reason, bypass grafting of the RCA may be worth considering since the development of right heart failure after LVAD placement is associated with high mortality [88]. Second, although unusual, some patients with severe coronary disease may continue to experience angina post-LVAD implantation. Finally, in the event of a device failure, native heart function will be less than optimal if the myocardium is significantly ischemic. For technical reasons, some have advised placing the proximal anastomosis of the saphenous vein graft on the LVAD outflow graft, rather than the aorta.

5.4.6   Other Concomitant Cardiac Surgery

Previously recognized atrial and/or ventricular septal defects or those identified at the time of LVAD placement should be repaired simultaneously with the implant to avoid right to left shunting which may occur as a consequence of right heart failure and/or decreased left-sided pressures. The same is true for any TEE recognized PFOs [89–91]. Finally, ligation or closure of the left atrial appendage could be considered in patients with atrial fibrillation.

5.5 Postoperative Considerations

Even if the surgery, recovery, and rehabilitation proceed uneventfully, unexpected postoperative problems may develop. The most serious of these are pump thrombosis, cerebrovascular complications, infections, and valvular abnormalities. How to handle some of these issues during the preoperative and intraoperative period was partially reviewed above. How to address these issues and reduce the likelihood of occurrence in the postoperative period is reviewed below.

5.5.1 Pump Thrombosis

Even with an acceptable flow rate and appropriate anticoagulation, pump thrombosis will occur. The actual percentage will vary from device to device and upon the anticoagulation protocol used. In general, the rate is less than 5 % in most trials regardless of whether the pump is an axial flow pump or a centrifugal flow pump [92]. Whether the clot is forming in situ or is being sucked in from the ventricle (or atrium) is often not clear. How axial and centrifugal pumps handle the clot may differ as well.

Russell presented a retrospective review of over 700 HM II patients (1,000 patient-years) in 2011. Twenty-six events were reported in 23 patients for an event per patient-year rate of 0.03. By multivariate analysis, risk factors for pump thrombosis included age >65 years, albumin <3.3 mg/dL, female gender, and ischemic etiology [77].

Making the diagnosis of pump thrombosis (not outflow graft or inflow graft obstruction) is not always easy. With most axial and centrifugal pumps one sets the speed. The computer algorithms then calculate the flow based upon some hydrodynamic assumptions and based upon the measured power consumption. When a thrombus develops on a rotor the amount of power needed to turn the impeller at the set rate will increase. The system interprets the increased power consumption as a reflection of increased flow. Therefore, any evidence of increasing power and increasing flow (or "pseudo-flow" as there really is not an increase in flow actually occurring) in the presence of clinical or laboratory signs of hemolysis (such as an elevation of the LDH or increase in plasma free hemoglobin) should raise the possibility of pump thrombosis [93, 94]. Unfortunately, not all VAD systems provide data in real time.

Assessing LV cavity size at various RPM settings has been shown to help diagnose/confirm pump thrombosis in axial flow devices. Similar data has not been demonstrated for centrifugal flow devices (again probably due to the different HQ curves). This process is colloquially known as "ramp testing" and is being used with increasing frequency to allow for earlier intervention in the hope of improving clinical outcomes [95].

If making the diagnosis of pump thrombosis is difficult, figuring out how to best treat the problem is even more problematic. When this complication occurred in the past with the MicroMed DeBakey pump, intravenous thrombolytic therapy was advised. The safety of thrombolytics, however, has not been established given the theoretical possibility that lysed clot might propagate downstream and result in an embolic cerebrovascular accident (CVA) [96]. Other approaches have been tried with variable success rates including intraventricular thrombolytics which appear to have an approximately 50 % success rate [97]. Given the risks and the relatively low efficacy, thrombolytic therapy is not normally considered first-line treatment. Instead, pump thrombosis or suspected pump thrombosis is treated by enhancing the degree of anticoagulation usually through the addition of unfractionated heparin. Surprisingly, this relatively simple intervention does seem to work a good percentage of the time. For those cases in which the VAD parameters (power consumption) and/or the biological markers (LDH, plasma free hemoglobin, and BNP) fail to return to normal, device exchange (perhaps using a subcostal incision) needs to be considered, probably sooner rather than later [98, 99]. In most cases the explanation for the pump thrombosis is never established. Sometimes, however, the problem is technical and can be attributed to obstruction to inflow due to a shift in cannula position. In such cases, replacement of the VAD without changing the angulations or location of the VAD may result in the same problem a few months later.

5.5.2 Infection Prophylaxis

Device-related infections remain a significant complication of LVAD therapy. Infections may be further classified as preimplantation, postimplantation, and post-transplantation [100]. The usual sites of infection with assist devices are bloodstream, driveline, mediastinum, and the device itself (although this is less frequent with the axial and centrifugal pumps as compared to the now "retired" HeartMate XVE). The typical offending organisms are those that form biofilms such as staphylococcus, enterococcus, corynebacterium, pseudomonas, and candida [101].

Preoperative issues such as obesity, malnutrition/debilitation, and active infections undoubtedly affect postoperative infection risk. The presence of these comorbidities does not necessarily preclude device implantation; however, it does make it incumbent upon the evaluating team to extend all efforts to mitigate the risk. One simple intervention is to ensure that all old intravenous lines (including the PICC) be removed at least 24 h preoperatively. New lines should be placed in the operating room and lines should be changed postoperatively in accordance with CDC guidelines for indwelling catheters. As well, standardized antibiotic protocols should be followed. One representative example of a standardized protocol (assuming normal renal function) is set forth below. Protocols need to be adjusted for the institution's local flora and sensitivities:

1. Vancomycin 15 mg/kg IV 30–60 min prior to skin incision, then q12 h×48–72 h
2. Levofloxacin 500 mg or Cefepime 1 g IV 1 h prior to skin incision, then q24 h×48–72 h
3. Rifampin 600 mg IV 1 to 2 hours pre-op, then q24 h×48–72 h
4. Fluconazole 400 mg IV pre-op then q24 h×48–72 h
5. Bactroban applied to each nostril the evening before surgery

Specific evidence-based interventions include preparation of the surgical site with an appropriate antiseptic agent, proper sterilization and disinfection of equipment, minimizing traffic in the operating room, and use of appropriate ventilation systems. Other approaches address modifiable patient-related factors such as tight perioperative blood glucose control for patients with diabetes. Rehabilitation and nutrition play an important role in immunity and wound healing [102].

Postoperatively, infections are defined as VAD specific (pump, cannulae, pocket, and driveline), VAD-related (endocarditis, bacteremia, and mediastinitis), and non-VAD (urinary tract infection, Clostridium difficile colitis, cholecystitis, pneumonia, etc.) [100, 103]. Major and minor criteria have been developed to help clinicians categorize the infection [100]. Should the patient develop an infection, standard antibiotic therapy is utilized. If the source of the infection is the driveline, frequent dressing changes are used to ensure that the exit site remains dry. Some centers may wash the site with a gentamicin scrub. Others use biopatches impregnated with chlorhexidine. All centers ensure strict immobilization of the driveline. A study showed that the percutaneous site infections (PSI) occur in approximately 19 % of continuous-flow LVAD recipients by 12 months after implant [104]. Young age was the only predictor of PSI. It is generally accepted that the development of a PSI will adversely affect survival with sepsis being the most common cause of death (26.1 %) [104].

5.5.3 *Late Postoperative Bleeding*

Bleeding issues related to the HeartMate II device were identified fairly early in the HM II trial [105]. The investigators noted that patients were experiencing higher rates of GI bleeding than might ordinarily be expected given the degree of anticoagulation [106, 107]. Extensive analysis was performed and it was eventually concluded that the HM II (and perhaps all devices with high shear forces) was causing the loss of high molecular weight von Willebrand Factor (vWF) multimers (HMWM) [108, 109]. Seemingly, the shear forces unravel the vWF, thereby allowing ADAMTS-13 to cleave it. In fact, one study showed that although 75 % of all device recipients had normal levels of high molecular weight multimers preoperatively, most of them had a moderate to severe loss of HMWM by day 7 and by day 30 100 % had a loss of HMWM [110]. Presumably, this loss of HMWM is somehow associated with the development of occult and/or intermittent GI bleeding (often due to arteriovenous malformations—otherwise known as Heyde syndrome when seen in patients with chronic aortic stenosis).

The GI bleeding rate (defined as the need for a transfusion of >2 units PRBC) for the Thoratec HM II pump appears to be higher than the GI bleeding rate for the HeartWare HVAD [111]. Moreover, the rate of GI bleeding seems to vary greatly from institution to institution for reasons which are not entirely clear. It may or may not be related to the RPM set point [112]. The generally reported rate is about 20–25 % at 12 months [107, 113]. Discontinuing anticoagulation is the normal response to bleeding and would seem to be the logical response in LVAD patients as well, the clotting risk notwithstanding. Other options for treating GI bleeding in LVAD recipients include cauterization, cryoprecipitate, von Willebrand factor concentrates, DDAVP (which releases endothelial stores of vWF), Humate-P, and perhaps Novoseven [114]. Most experts advise strongly against the use of prothrombin complex concentrates which are known to cause thrombosis even in "normal" individuals. Likewise, the use of thalidomide (which may be a reasonable treatment for angiodysplasia or AV malformations) also poses a thrombotic risk and would probably be a less than ideal intervention in LVAD patients (especially if the warfarin was discontinued). Use of thalidomide requires that the physician receive special education/certification. Potentially safer (albeit unproven) options include subcutaneous octreotide and oral estrogen conjugates [114–116].

5.5.4 Cerebrovascular Events

The development of a cerebrovascular event after LVAD implantation is a devastating complication [7, 117]. The incidence of CVA after LVAD placement reportedly ranges from 8 to 25 % depending upon the device and definition of a CVA [118, 119]. An analysis of the INTERMACS database, which includes pulsatile-flow and continuous-flow devices, also reported that a neurological complication (NC) was one of the leading causes of death [26].

Data from the 140 patient ADVANCE BTT HeartWare HVAD trial demonstrated an ischemic CVA rate of 7.5 % (0.09 per patient-year (PPY)) and hemorrhagic CVA rate of 7.8 % (0.09 PPY) [120]. In response to the relatively high CVA rates, the company redesigned the pump by sintering the inflow conduit, enlarging the coring tool, and changing the recommended aspirin dosage from 81 to 325 mg daily. Interestingly, this decreased the rate of pump thrombosis from 0.06 to 0.025 PPY but produced only minimal reductions on the rates of ischemic and hemorrhagic strokes. Most ischemic strokes occurred in the early perioperative period and approximately 75 % recovered with minimal deficits. For comparison, the published ischemic stroke rate for the 281 patient Thoratec HeartMate II BTT trial was 0.09 PPY and the hemorrhagic stroke rate was 0.05 PPY [113].

In axial flow pumps, cerebrovascular events are said to be increased by four to nine times during the 14 days window around an episode of a systemic infection. Driveline infections, in contrast, are not typically associated with an increased risk.

Exactly why the risk of a CVA is increased by systemic infection is not clear. One thing to consider, however, is that high-dose broad-spectrum antibiotics by altering gut flora indirectly affect warfarin metabolism. Perhaps this alteration results in higher INRs and a higher CVA rate. Obviously, this is all highly speculative. Nonetheless, it highlights the importance of maintaining patients in an infection-free state.

In a recent review of 307 consecutive patients who underwent LVAD surgery (167 HeartMate I and 140 HeartMate II devices) at Columbia University Medical Center between November 2000 and December 2010, the authors demonstrated that overall frequency of neurologic complications including TIA after LVAD placement was 14.0 % and that of ischemic/hemorrhagic CVA 11.4 % [121]. No statistical difference was noted between patients implanted with the HeartMate XVE and the HeartMate II. A history of a CVA and the presence of a postoperative infection were independently associated with development of NCs after LVAD placement [121].

5.5.5 Valvular Issues

Valvular problems, which were a nonissue with the HeartMate XVE (due to the short duration of support), have become an increasingly significant problem for the newer devices. The most frequent valvular problem encountered is aortic insufficiency (AI) [122]. While most LVAD recipients are screened preoperatively for this valvular lesion it appears that the problem is now developing de novo after device placement [123]. Predicting who will develop AI is difficult. Anecdotally, however, it does appear to develop beyond 12 months and more frequently in small patients, elderly patients, and women. Whether there is an association with pump speed is not known. Likewise, it is not known whether patients whose valve leaflets remain closed (due to high RPM related LV chamber emptying) are at higher risk than patients whose valve leaflets open intermittently. One thing is certain—leaflet fusion and secondary leaflet distortion will develop in some patients resulting in signs and symptoms of recurrent CHF. Next-generation devices are likely to incorporate algorithms designed to automatically ensure that the aortic valve opens intermittently. Until then, however, may be of some benefit to set the device at 9M RPM at which the aortic valve opens intermittently.

5.5.6 Blood Pressure Control

One other potential explanation for the increased rate of postoperative neurologic complications is unrecognized hypertension. As these devices pump continuously throughout the entire cardiac cycle, normal pulsatile flow is absent. Consistently recording an accurate blood pressure with a standard sphygmomanometer is not always easy [123]. Moreover, the mean is never measured. The use of a Doppler cuff should be encouraged. Unfortunately, the manufacturer of the most commonly used device (Terumo) recently discontinued distribution of the Doppler cuff in the United States. Ideally, the mean arterial blood pressure should be maintained between 70 and 80 mmHg and should not exceed 90 mmHg [124].

Blood pressure control is best achieved using standard oral antihypertensive medications. Management of hypertension by adjusting the RPM of the VAD is not recommended.

5.6 Conclusion

As the number of patients with end-stage heart failure increases while the number of donor hearts remains static, the only realistic option for the foreseeable future remains mechanical circulatory support. As such, one can assume that this technology will become more widely used as the years progress. Given the expense associated with long-term mechanical support, it is incumbent upon all practitioners to ensure that not only are the appropriate candidates being identified but that they are identified as early as possible in order to optimize their preoperative condition and improve their short- and long-term survival and quality of life. The recommendations set forth in this chapter should be considered guidelines only and are subject to change and modification as additional large-scale randomized trials shed new light on the field of mechanical circulatory support.

References

1. Stehlik J et al. The registry of the international society for heart and lung transplantation: twenty-ninth adult heart transplant report–2012. J Heart Lung Transplant. 2012;31(10):1052–64.
2. Taylor DO et al. Registry of the international society for heart and lung transplantation: twenty-fourth official adult heart transplant report–2007. J Heart Lung Transplant. 2007;26(8):769–81.
3. Dennis CC. The use of pump oxygenator support in heart failure. J Oslo City Hosp. 1961;11:107–8.
4. Spencer FC et al. Assisted circulation for cardiac failure following intracardiac surgery with cardiopulmonary bypass. J Thorac Cardiovasc Surg. 1965;49:56–73.
5. Bernhard WF et al. An appraisal of blood trauma and blood-prosthetic interface during left ventricular bypass in the calf and humans. Ann Thorac Surg. 1978;26(5):427–37.
6. Norman JC et al. Intracorporeal (abdominal) left ventricular assist devices or partial artificial hearts: a five-year clinical experience. Arch Surg. 1981;116(11):1441–5.
7. Rose EA et al. Long-term use of a left ventricular assist device for end-stage heart failure. N Engl J Med. 2001;345(20):1435–43.
8. Barge-Caballero E et al. Usefulness of the INTERMACS scale for predicting outcomes after urgent heart transplantation. Rev Esp Cardiol. 2011;64(3):193–200.
9. Boyle AJ et al. Clinical outcomes for continuous-flow left ventricular assist device patients stratified by pre-operative INTERMACS classification. J Heart Lung Transplant. 2011;30(4):402–7.
10. Alba AC et al. Usefulness of the INTERMACS scale to predict outcomes after mechanical assist device implantation. J Heart Lung Transplant. 2009;28(8):827–33.

11. Slaughter MS et al. Clinical management of continuous-flow left ventricular assist devices in advanced heart failure. J Heart Lung Transplant. 2010;29(4 Suppl):S1–39.

12. Miller LW, Guglin M. Patient selection for ventricular assist devices: a moving target. J Am Coll Cardiol. 2013;61(12):1209–21.

13. Hunt SA et al. 2009 Focused update incorporated into the ACC/AHA 2005 guidelines for the diagnosis and management of heart failure in adults. A report of the American College of Cardiology Foundation/American Heart Association Task Force on Practice Guidelines developed in collaboration with the International Society for Heart and Lung Transplantation. J Am Coll Cardiol. 2009;53(15):e1–90.

14. Lindenfeld J et al. HFSA 2010 comprehensive heart failure practice guideline. J Card Fail. 2010;16(6):e1–194.

15. Dickstein K et al. 2010 focused update of ESC guidelines on device therapy in heart failure: an update of the 2008 ESC Guidelines for the diagnosis and treatment of acute and chronic heart failure and the 2007 ESC Guidelines for cardiac and resynchronization therapy. Developed with the special contribution of the Heart Failure Association and the European Heart Rhythm Association. Eur J Heart Fail. 2010;12(11):1143–53.

16. McMurray JJ et al. ESC guidelines for the diagnosis and treatment of acute and chronic heart failure 2012: the task force for the diagnosis and treatment of acute and chronic heart failure 2012 of the European Society of Cardiology. Developed in collaboration with the heart failure association (HFA) of the ESC. Eur J Heart Fail. 2012;14(8):803–69.

17. Peura JL et al. Recommendations for the use of mechanical circulatory support: device strategies and patient selection: a scientific statement from the American Heart Association. Circulation. 2012;126(22):2648–67.

18. Rector TS et al. Use of left ventricular assist devices as destination therapy in end-stage congestive heart failure: a systematic review. VA-ESP Project #09-009; 2012.

19. Oz MC et al. Selection criteria for placement of left ventricular assist devices. Am Heart J. 1995;129(1):173–7.

20. Rao V et al. Revised screening scale to predict survival after insertion of a left ventricular assist device. J Thorac Cardiovasc Surg. 2003;125(4):855–62.

21. Lietz K et al. Outcomes of left ventricular assist device implantation as destination therapy in the post-REMATCH era: implications for patient selection. Circulation. 2007;116(5): 497–505.

22. Schaffer JM et al. Evaluation of risk indices in continuous-flow left ventricular assist device patients. Ann Thorac Surg. 2009;88(6):1889–96.

23. Cowger J et al. Predicting survival in patients receiving continuous flow left ventricular assist devices: the HeartMate II risk score. J Am Coll Cardiol. 2013;61(3):313–21.

24. Matthews JC et al. The right ventricular failure risk score a pre-operative tool for assessing the risk of right ventricular failure in left ventricular assist device candidates. J Am Coll Cardiol. 2008;51(22):2163–72.

25. Fitzpatrick 3rd JR et al. Risk score derived from pre-operative data analysis predicts the need for biventricular mechanical circulatory support. J Heart Lung Transplant. 2008;27(12):1286–92.

26. Kirklin JK et al. Second INTERMACS annual report: more than 1,000 primary left ventricular assist device implants. J Heart Lung Transplant. 2010;29(1):1–10.

27. Kormos RL et al. Right ventricular failure in patients with the HeartMate II continuous-flow left ventricular assist device: incidence, risk factors, and effect on outcomes. J Thorac Cardiovasc Surg. 2010;139(5):1316–24.

28. Korabathina R et al. The pulmonary artery pulsatility index identifies severe right ventricular dysfunction in acute inferior myocardial infarction. Catheter Cardiovasc Interv. 2012;80(4):593–600.

29. Morrison DA. Guilt by association: after enhanced interrogation, the data yield a confession. Catheter Cardiovasc Interv. 2012;80(4):601–2.

30. Grant AD et al. Independent and incremental role of quantitative right ventricular evaluation for the prediction of right ventricular failure after left ventricular assist device implantation. J Am Coll Cardiol. 2012;60(6):521–8.

31. Wang L et al. Predicting right ventricular failure in patients undergoing ventricular assist device implantation using speckle tracking imaging. J Am Coll Cardiol. 2012;59(13s1):E1019. doi:10.1016/S0735-1097(12)61020-1.
32. Wang L et al. Pre-operative velocity vector imaging to predict the need for right ventricular support in patients undergoing left ventricular assist device implantation. J Heart Lung Transplant. 2013;32(4):S273–4.
33. Munoz-Garcia AJ et al. Survival and predictive factors of mortality after 30 days in patients treated with percutaneous implantation of the CoreValve aortic prosthesis. Am Heart J. 2012;163(2):288–94.
34. Dewey TM. Frailty scores and the writing on the wall. JACC Cardiovasc Interv. 2012;5(5):497–8.
35. Flint KM et al. Frailty and the selection of patients for destination therapy left ventricular assist device. Circ Heart Fail. 2012;5(2):286–93.
36. Heise D et al. Recombinant activated factor VII (Novo7) in patients with ventricular assist devices: case report and review of the current literature. J Cardiothorac Surg. 2007;2:47.
37. Fries D et al. Coagulation monitoring and management of anticoagulation during cardiac assist device support. Ann Thorac Surg. 2003;76(5):1593–7.
38. Zucker MJ et al. Cardiac transplantation and/or mechanical circulatory support device placement using heparin anti-coagulation in the presence of acute heparin-induced thrombocytopenia. J Heart Lung Transplant. 2010;29(1):53–60.
39. Kiernan MS et al. Right ventricular failure in patients with continuous-flow left ventricular assist devices: incidence and risk factors from INTERMACS. J Heart Lung Transplant. 2012;31(4):S110–1.
40. Cleveland Jr JC et al. Survival after biventricular assist device implantation: an analysis of the Interagency Registry for Mechanically Assisted Circulatory Support database. J Heart Lung Transplant. 2011;30(8):862–9.
41. Kirklin JK et al. Fifth INTERMACS annual report: risk factor analysis from more than 6,000 mechanical circulatory support patients. J Heart Lung Transplant. 2013;32(2):141–56.
42. Lainez R et al. Right ventricular function and left ventricular assist device placement: clinical considerations and outcomes. Ochsner J. 2010;10(4):241–4.
43. Drakos SG et al. Risk factors predictive of right ventricular failure after left ventricular assist device implantation. Am J Cardiol. 2010;105(7):1030–5.
44. Ochiai Y et al. Predictors of severe right ventricular failure after implantable left ventricular assist device insertion: analysis of 245 patients. Circulation. 2002;106(12 Suppl 1): I198–202.
45. Fukamachi K et al. Preoperative risk factors for right ventricular failure after implantable left ventricular assist device insertion. Ann Thorac Surg. 1999;68(6):2181–4.
46. Meineri M et al. Right ventricular failure after LVAD implantation: prevention and treatment. Best Pract Res Clin Anaesthesiol. 2012;26(2):217–29.
47. Puhlman M. Continuous-flow left ventricular assist device and the right ventricle. AACN Adv Crit Care. 2012;23(1):86–90.
48. John R et al. Right ventricular failure–a continuing problem in patients with left ventricular assist device support. J Cardiovasc Transl Res. 2010;3(6):604–11.
49. Henderson KK et al. Physiological replacement of T3 improves left ventricular function in an animal model of myocardial infarction-induced congestive heart failure. Circ Heart Fail. 2009;2(3):243–52.
50. Uriel N et al. Thyroid deficiency is common in advanced heart failure and associated with increased operative mortality after assist device implantation. J Heart Lung Transplant. 2010;28(2):S25.
51. Neragi-Miandoab S et al. Right ventricular dysfunction following continuous flow left ventricular assist device placement in 51 patients: predicators and outcomes. J Cardiothorac Surg. 2012;7:60.
52. Morgan JA et al. Impact of continuous-flow left ventricular assist device support on right ventricular function. J Heart Lung Transplant. 2013;32(4):398–403.

53. Potapov E et al. Inhaled nitric oxide after left ventricular assist device implantation: a prospective, randomized, double-blind, multicenter, placebo-controlled trial. J Heart Lung Transplant. 2011;30(8):870–8.
54. Macdonald PS et al. Adjunctive use of inhaled nitric oxide during implantation of a left ventricular assist device. J Heart Lung Transplant. 1998;17(3):312–6.
55. Chang JC et al. Hemodynamic effect of inhaled nitric oxide in dilated cardiomyopathy patients on LVAD support. ASAIO J. 1997;43(5):M418–21.
56. Radovancevic B et al. Nitric oxide versus prostaglandin E1 for reduction of pulmonary hypertension in heart transplant candidates. J Heart Lung Transplant. 2005;24(6):690–5.
57. Murali S et al. Reversibility of pulmonary hypertension in congestive heart failure patients evaluated for cardiac transplantation: comparative effects of various pharmacologic agents. Am Heart J. 1991;122(5):1375–81.
58. Tedford RJ et al. PDE5A inhibitor treatment of persistent pulmonary hypertension after mechanical circulatory support. Circ Heart Fail. 2008;1(4):213–9.
59. Estep JD et al. The role of echocardiography and other imaging modalities in patients with left ventricular assist devices. JACC Cardiovasc Imaging. 2010;3(10):1049–64.
60. Rich JD. Right ventricular failure in patients with left ventricular assist devices. Cardiol Clin. 2012;30(2):291–302.
61. Baumwol J et al. Right heart failure and "failure to thrive" after left ventricular assist device: clinical predictors and outcomes. J Heart Lung Transplant. 2011;30(8):888–95.
62. Cohn WE. New tools and techniques to facilitate off-pump left ventricular assist device implantation. Tex Heart Inst J. 2010;37(5):559–61.
63. Feldman D et al. The 2013 International Society for Heart and Lung Transplantation Guidelines for mechanical circulatory support: executive summary. J Heart Lung Transplant. 2013;32(2):157–87.
64. Tector AJ et al. Transition from cardiopulmonary bypass to the HeartMate left ventricular assist device. Ann Thorac Surg. 1998;65(3):643–6.
65. John R et al. Low thromboembolic risk for patients with the Heartmate II left ventricular assist device. J Thorac Cardiovasc Surg. 2008;136(5):1318–23.
66. Slaughter MS et al. Post-operative heparin may not be required for transitioning patients with a HeartMate II left ventricular assist system to long-term warfarin therapy. J Heart Lung Transplant. 2010;29(6):616–24.
67. Menon AK et al. Low stroke rate and few thrombo-embolic events after HeartMate II implantation under mild anticoagulation. Eur J Cardiothorac Surg. 2012;42(2):319–23. discussion 323.
68. Morshuis M et al. A modified technique for implantation of the HeartWare left ventricular assist device when using bivalirudin anticoagulation in patients with acute heparin-induced thrombocytopenia. Interact Cardiovasc Thorac Surg. 2013;17(2):225–6.
69. Awad H et al. Thrombosis during off pump LVAD placement in a patient with heparin induced thrombocytopenia using bivalirudin. J Cardiothorac Surg. 2013;8(1):115.
70. Schmitz ML et al. Management of a pediatric patient on the Berlin Heart Excor ventricular assist device with argatroban after heparin-induced thrombocytopenia. ASAIO J. 2008;54(5):546–7.
71. Takahama T, Kanai F, Onishi K. Anticoagulation during use of a left ventricular assist device. ASAIO J. 2000;46(3):354–7.
72. Takahama T et al. Ideal anticoagulation for use with a left ventricular assist device. ASAIO J. 1995;41(3):M779–82.
73. Christiansen S et al. Anticoagulative management of patients requiring left ventricular assist device implantation and suffering from heparin-induced thrombocytopenia type II. Ann Thorac Surg. 2000;69(3):774–7.
74. Pereira NL et al. Discontinuation of antithrombotic therapy for a year or more in patients with continuous-flow left ventricular assist devices. Interact Cardiovasc Thorac Surg. 2010;11(4):503–5.
75. Stern DR et al. Increased incidence of gastrointestinal bleeding following implantation of the HeartMate II LVAD. J Card Surg. 2010;25(3):352–6.

76. Rossi M et al. What is the optimal anticoagulation in patients with a left ventricular assist device? Interact Cardiovasc Thorac Surg. 2012;15(4):733–40.
77. Russell SD et al. Risk of bleeding and stroke in 700 HeartMate II LVAD outpatients. J Heart Lung Transplant. 2011;30(4):S66.
78. Boyle AJ et al. Low thromboembolism and pump thrombosis with the HeartMate II left ventricular assist device: analysis of outpatient anti-coagulation. J Heart Lung Transplant. 2009;28(9):881–7.
79. Dranishnikov N et al. Simultaneous aortic valve replacement in left ventricular assist device recipients: single-center experience. Int J Artif Organs. 2012;35(7):489–94.
80. Feldman CM et al. Management of aortic insufficiency with continuous flow left ventricular assist devices: bioprosthetic valve replacement. J Heart Lung Transplant. 2006;25(12): 1410–2.
81. Rao V et al. Surgical management of valvular disease in patients requiring left ventricular assist device support. Ann Thorac Surg. 2001;71(5):1448–53.
82. Pal JD et al. Low operative mortality with implantation of a continuous-flow left ventricular assist device and impact of concurrent cardiac procedures. Circulation. 2009;120(11 Suppl):S215–9.
83. Nahumi DB et al. Aortic insufficiency and clinical outcomes in patients undergoing aortic valve procedures at the time of continuous flow left ventricular assist device implantation. J Heart Lung Transplant. 2013;32(4):S278.
84. Moazami N et al. Inflow valve regurgitation during left ventricular assist device support may interfere with reverse ventricular remodeling. Ann Thorac Surg. 1998;65(3):628–31.
85. Holman WL et al. Influence of longer term left ventricular assist device support on valvular regurgitation. ASAIO J. 1994;40(3):M454–9.
86. Westaby S. Tricuspid regurgitation in left ventricular assist device patients. Eur J Cardiothorac Surg. 2012;41(1):217–8.
87. Piacentino 3rd V et al. Clinical impact of concomitant tricuspid valve procedures during left ventricular assist device implantation. Ann Thorac Surg. 2011;92(4):1414–8. discussion 1418–9.
88. Potapov EV et al. Revascularization of the occluded right coronary artery during left ventricular assist device implantation. J Heart Lung Transplant. 2001;20(8):918–22.
89. Bartoli CR et al. Percutaneous closure of a patent foramen ovale to prevent paradoxical thromboembolism in a patient with a continuous-flow LVAD. J Invasive Cardiol. 2013;25(3): 154–6.
90. Loforte A et al. Transcatheter closure of patent foramen ovale for hypoxemia during left ventricular assist device support. J Card Surg. 2012;27(4):528–9.
91. Kapur NK et al. Percutaneous closure of patent foramen ovale for refractory hypoxemia after HeartMate II left ventricular assist device placement. J Invasive Cardiol. 2007;19(9):E268–70.
92. Sheikh FH et al. HeartMate(R) II continuous-flow left ventricular assist system. Expert Rev Med Devices. 2011;8(1):11–21.
93. Meyer AL et al. Thrombus formation in a HeartMate II left ventricular assist device. J Thorac Cardiovasc Surg. 2008;135(1):203–4.
94. Bhamidipati CM et al. Early thrombus in a HeartMate II left ventricular assist device: a potential cause of hemolysis and diagnostic dilemma. J Thorac Cardiovasc Surg. 2010;140(1):e7–8.
95. Uriel N et al. Development of a novel echocardiography ramp test for speed optimization and diagnosis of device thrombosis in continuous-flow left ventricular assist devices: the Columbia ramp study. J Am Coll Cardiol. 2012;60(18):1764–75.
96. Muthiah K et al. Thrombolysis for suspected intrapump thrombosis in patients with continuous flow centrifugal left ventricular assist device. Artif Organs. 2013;37(3):313–8.
97. Kiernan MS et al. Management of HeartWare left ventricular assist device thrombosis using intracavitary thrombolytics. J Thorac Cardiovasc Surg. 2011;142(3):712–4.
98. Moazami N et al. Pump replacement for left ventricular assist device failure can be done safely and is associated with low mortality. Ann Thorac Surg. 2013;95(2):500–5.
99. Goldstein D et al. Algorithm for the diagnosis and management of suspected pump thrombus. J Heart Lung Transplant. 2013;32:667–70.

100. Hannan MM et al. Working formulation for the standardization of definitions of infections in patients using ventricular assist devices. J Heart Lung Transplant. 2011;30(4):375–84.
101. Acharya MN et al. Tsui, what is the optimum antibiotic prophylaxis in patients undergoing implantation of a left ventricular assist device? Interact Cardiovasc Thorac Surg. 2012;14(2):209–14.
102. Califano S et al. Left ventricular assist device-associated infections. Infect Dis Clin North Am. 2012;26(1):77–87.
103. Guerrero-Miranda C et al. Classification of ventricular assist device infections according to ISHLT formulation and device generation. J Heart Lung Transplant. 2012;31(4):S21.
104. Goldstein DJ et al. Continuous-flow devices and percutaneous site infections: clinical outcomes. J Heart Lung Transplant. 2012;31(11):1151–7.
105. Park SJ et al. Outcomes in advanced heart failure patients with left ventricular assist devices for destination therapy. Circ Heart Fail. 2012;5(2):241–8.
106. Islam S et al. Left ventricular assist devices and gastrointestinal bleeding: a narrative review of case reports and case series. Clin Cardiol. 2013;36(4):190–200.
107. Morgan JA et al. Gastrointestinal bleeding with the HeartMate II left ventricular assist device. J Heart Lung Transplant. 2012;31(7):715–8.
108. Klovaite J et al. Severely impaired von Willebrand factor-dependent platelet aggregation in patients with a continuous-flow left ventricular assist device (HeartMate II). J Am Coll Cardiol. 2009;53(23):2162–7.
109. Malehsa D et al. Acquired von Willebrand syndrome after exchange of the HeartMate XVE to the HeartMate II ventricular assist device. Eur J Cardiothorac Surg. 2009;35(6):1091–3.
110. Crow S et al. Acquired von Willebrand syndrome in continuous-flow ventricular assist device recipients. Ann Thorac Surg. 2010;90(4):1263–9. discussion 1269.
111. Hosseini MT et al. Comparison of left ventricular geometry after HeartMate II and HeartWare left ventricular assist device implantation. J Cardiothorac Surg. 2013;8:31.
112. Patel SR et al. Gastrointestinal bleeding is not associated with pump speed and aortic valve opening in patients supported with the HeartMate II LVAD. J Heart Lung Transplant. 2012;31(4):S34.
113. Pagani FD et al. Extended mechanical circulatory support with a continuous-flow rotary left ventricular assist device. J Am Coll Cardiol. 2009;54(4):312–21.
114. Suarez J et al. Mechanisms of bleeding and approach to patients with axial-flow left ventricular assist devices. Circ Heart Fail. 2011;4(6):779–84.
115. Hayes HM et al. Management options to treat gastrointestinal bleeding in patients supported on rotary left ventricular assist devices: a single-center experience. Artif Organs. 2010;34(9): 703–6.
116. Aggarwal A et al. Incidence and management of gastrointestinal bleeding with continuous flow assist devices. Ann Thorac Surg. 2012;93(5):1534–40.
117. Nakajima I et al. Pre- and post-operative risk factors associated with cerebrovascular accidents in patients supported by left ventricular assist device. Single center's experience in Japan. Circ J. 2011;75(5):1138–46.
118. Slaughter MS et al. Advanced heart failure treated with continuous-flow left ventricular assist device. N Engl J Med. 2009;361(23):2241–51.
119. Tsukui H et al. Cerebrovascular accidents in patients with a ventricular assist device. J Thorac Cardiovasc Surg. 2007;134(1):114–23.
120. Aaronson KD et al. Use of an intrapericardial, continuous-flow, centrifugal pump in patients awaiting heart transplantation. Circulation. 2012;125(25):3191–200.
121. Kato TS et al. Pre-operative and post-operative risk factors associated with neurologic complications in patients with advanced heart failure supported by a left ventricular assist device. J Heart Lung Transplant. 2012;31(1):1–8.
122. Aggarwal A et al. The development of aortic insufficiency in continuous-flow left ventricular assist device-supported patients. Ann Thorac Surg. 2013;95(2):493–8.
123. Bejar NN et al. The prevalence of aortic insufficiency in patients maintained on continuous flow left ventricular assist devices. J Heart Lung Transplant. 2013;32(4):S278.
124. Coyle LA et al. Measurement of blood pressure during support with a continuous-flow left ventricular assist device in the outpatient setting. J Heart Lung Transplant. 2013;32(4):S235.

Chapter 6
Transplant Versus VAD: Evolving and Future Perspectives

Hiroo Takayama, Sunu Thomas, and Yoshifumi Naka

Abstract Continuous-flow left ventricular assist devices (CF-LVADs) have become an essential therapeutic option in the standard of care for patients with end-stage heart failure. Clinical outcomes continue to improve through better patient selection, surgical technique, and perioperative management. Current two-year survival rates could exceed 80 % with device support in selected patients, and this is comparable to that of cardiac transplantation. As such, there has been a proliferation in the number of patients receiving device therapy and the centers implanting them. Moreover, CF-LVADs may also provide a platform for innovative treatments, including regenerative and stem cell therapies, to promote functional recovery of the native heart. These advantageous features should encourage the use of CF-LVADs as a replacement for cardiac transplantation in patients with stage D heart failure. However, as compared to transplant, quality of life and device-related costs may be limiting factors. In this relatively nascent field, more clinical trial data, especially from long-term follow-up, will be necessary to evaluate the risks and benefits of durable device support. Ultimately, a head-to-head comparison between the two therapies may need to be considered to answer the inevitable question: *can CF-LVAD therapy replace cardiac transplantation as the preferred treatment for advanced heart disease*? In the current era, however, it is far more important to appreciate how both strategies may be complementary and under what circumstances, one obviates the other, in order to achieve the best clinical outcome for the patient with end-stage heart failure.

H. Takayama • Y. Naka (⊠)
Division of Cardiothoracic Surgery, Columbia University, 177 Fort Washington Ave, MHB 7-435, New York, NY 10032, USA
e-mail: yn33@columbia.edu

S. Thomas
Division of Cardiology, Columbia University, 177 Fort Washington Ave, MHB 7-435, New York, NY 10032, USA

S. Kyo (ed.), *Ventricular Assist Devices in Advanced-Stage Heart Failure*,
DOI 10.1007/978-4-431-54466-1_6, © Springer Japan 2014

Keywords Cardiac transplantation • Cost • Left ventricular assist device • Quality of life • Survival

6.1 Introduction

In the USA alone, more than six million patients suffer from heart failure. Over 600,000 new cases are diagnosed annually attesting to the epidemic gravity of this disease [1]. The current state of optimal pharmacotherapy entails a regimen of beta-blockers, angiotensin-converting enzyme inhibitors, angiotensin receptor blockers, and aldosterone antagonists to mitigate the neurohormonal cascade underlying pathophysiology of the heart failure state. Automated implantable cardiac defibrillators and cardiac resynchronization therapy are also implanted in eligible patients to improve both survival and overall quality of life in patients with chronic heart failure.

Despite developments in medical therapy that aim to prevent or delay the natural progression of myocardial dysfunction, the mortality rate amongst those with advanced disease is greater than 30 % per year [2]. For patients with stage D heart failure, characterized by advanced structural heart disease and refractory symptoms, hemodynamic tenuousness often necessitates the withdrawal of neurohormonal blockade to preserve an adequate blood pressure. Under such circumstances, symptoms may be improved with inotropic agents, albeit at the expense of an increased risk of mortality.

For eligible patients, cardiac transplantation remains the gold standard as a heart replacement therapy [3]. However, a significant deficit exists between the number of available donor hearts and heart failure patients in need. According to the International Society for Heart and Lung Transplantation (ISHLT), 3,892 cardiac transplants were performed in 2010 worldwide, representing only a fraction of those potential recipients actively wait-listed for a donor heart [4]. The number of cardiac transplants has remained constant over the last ten years despite the growing incidence of advanced heart disease in both globally and, specifically, in the USA, further compounding the limited options for patients with end-stage disease. Currently, 10–15 % of patients on the waiting list die before a suitable donor heart becomes available, with an additional 10–15 % being inactivated or frankly removed from the wait-list each year due to clinical deterioration rendering transplant surgery prohibitive [5]. With such constraints, the concept of cardiac transplantation as the "main stream" of treatment for end-stage heart failure must be questioned.

The inception of the artificial heart program by the National Heart, Lung and Blood Institute (NHLBI) in1964 enabled mechanical circulatory support device therapy to evolve into its current role with continuous-flow left ventricular assist device (CF-LVAD) technology as an additional heart replacement strategy for patients with end-stage heart failure [6]. The most recent Interagency Registry for Mechanically Assisted Circulatory Support (INTERMACS; a US registry for durable mechanical circulatory support device sponsored by the National Heart, Lung, and Blood Institute) report attests to over 6,000 VADs that have been implanted over the last 5 years reflecting the exponential growth mechanical support therapy amongst patients with end-stage heart failure. Currently, devices are used as univentricular (left vs. right) or biventricular support and as either a Bridge to Transplant (BTT) or Destination Therapy (DT) for those deemed transplant ineligible.

Ultimately, for those patients for whom reversal of heart failure is not possible, the question arises as to whether CF-LVAD therapy should be offered as the definitive strategy to patients with end-stage heart failure in lieu of a cardiac transplant. In this chapter, we will elaborate on this debate from the following perspectives: *patient selection, clinical outcomes including survival, adverse events, and quality of life, and cost-effectiveness.*

Understandably, an objective head-to-head comparison between cardiac transplant and CF-LVAD therapy is limited due to the absence of large-scale randomized clinical trials. In addition, long-term follow-up amongst CF-LVAD patients is also finite owing to the only recent Food and Drug Administration (FDA) approval for these devices as either BTT or DT strategies in the USA. However, data compiled from available clinical trials, institutional reports, and registries will provide insights from the experience with over 14,000 HeartMate II CF-LVADs (Thoratec Corp., Pleasanton, CA) that have been implanted worldwide as of May 2013.

Although other types of mechanical circulatory support devices, such as implantable biventricular assist device and total artificial heart, have also made progress, their clinical use and outcomes are yet far behind compared to those of CF-LVAD. The following sections mainly focus on comparing CF-LVAD with cardiac transplantation.

6.2 Patient Selection

For patients with end-stage heart failure, medical futility in resolving either symptoms or hemodynamic stability portends the poorest prognosis. Cardinal features that should prompt consideration for advanced therapies in such patients include hemodynamic intolerance of neurohormonal blockade, inotrope initiation, worsening end-organ dysfunction, frequent rehospitalizations, and poor predicted survival derived from cardiopulmonary exercise testing or risk calculators, such as the Seattle Heart Failure Risk Model.

Patient candidacy for either cardiac transplant or mechanical circulatory support is predicated on their perioperative mortality risk and consideration of comorbidities that would complicate survival and quality of life following initiation of an advanced therapy. Contraindications and surgical considerations are the predominant variables that distinguish both types of therapy and the patients to whom they may be offered.

Right ventricular function and pulmonary vasculature are major considerations in cardiac transplant and CF-LVAD decision-making. The presence of fixed pulmonary hypertension, typically defined as a transpulmonary gradient greater than 15 mmHg, pulmonary artery systolic pressure more than 60 mmHg, or a pulmonary vascular resistance higher than 6 Wood units not reversed with pulmonary vasodilatory testing, is an absolute contraindication for cardiac transplant [4]. Elevated pulmonary pressures predispose the donor heart to right ventricular failure and increased overall mortality risk. On the contrary, for patients with biventricular failure and normal or low pulmonary pressures, cardiac transplantation is an ideal strategy. However, the thought process becomes completely opposite for those under consideration for mechanical circulatory support. While the left ventricle is supported by a CF-LVAD, the device is preload dependent and, therefore, dependent on right ventricular function to ensure adequate left ventricular filling. High pulmonary artery pressure rather ensures reliable right ventricular function; whereas low pressure (with known biventricular failure/high CVP) is a manifestation of impaired right ventricular function. Numerous strategies including risk scores [7–9] and echocardiographic parameters [10] have been considered to assess the risk of developing right ventricular failure following LVAD placement. In the absence of a cardiac transplant, such patients require biventricular support either via a total artificial heart or the use of univentricular assist devices implanted into both right and left ventricles (or atria).

However, other conditions that would deny transplant consideration including recent malignancy, chronic renal failure (>2.0 mg/dL) with proteinuria, irreversible hepatic or pulmonary disease, and active systemic disease are not necessarily prohibitive for CF-LVAD therapy. In addition, sensitization due to the presence of circulating antibodies that limit donor availability, prolong wait-list times, and increase the risk of cardiac allograft rejection does not deter consideration for mechanical circulatory support. Patients in refractory cardiogenic shock are only salvaged with a device therapy because transplant assessment and identification of a suitable donor heart will not be completed in time.

Unlike a cardiac transplant that provides structural replacement of the patient's heart, the benefit with CF-LVAD therapy is derived from its hemodynamic support of the left ventricle. As such, the specific details related to the structure and function of the native heart must be accounted for prior to CF-LVAD placement that would otherwise not apply to cardiac transplant. In cases of restrictive cardiomyopathies, such as cardiac amyloidosis, small ventricular chamber size may be prohibitive for CF-LVAD inflow cannula placement and may further predispose to suction events. The presence of valvular disease may require surgical correction, which may increase cardiopulmonary bypass time and related intraoperative mortality risk although this conceptual concern does not seem applicable in our experience [11, 12]. As current generation devices require both antiplatelet and anticoagulant regimens and may predispose a patient to acquired von Willebrand disease, hypercoagulable states and predisposition to bleeding may further increase the associated morbidity and mortality with device-based therapy.

While there may be specific clinical circumstances in which cardiac transplant may be the preferred choice or vice versa, it is more important to recognize that two therapies concordantly contribute to improved clinical outcome. For example, patients with elevated pulmonary vascular resistance, which otherwise precludes the patient from receiving cardiac transplantation, can be bridged with LVAD therapy and undergo subsequent successful transplantation [13].

6.3   Survival

6.3.1   Cardiac Transplantation

The survival rate with cardiac transplantation has been relatively stable in the last two decades. Figure 6.1 shows the survival curve in the ISHLT registry [4]. In the UNOS registry, another large registry from the USA, the median survival for 43,906 heart transplants was approximately 9 years. At 20 years the survival rate continued to decline to reach <10 %. Seven-year survival rates for heart transplant recipients transplanted between 1998–1994, 1995–2000, and 2000–2007 were 59, 62, and 65 %, respectively [14]. Current post-transplant survival rate at 1, 2, 5, and 10 years is approximately 90, 80, 70, and 50 %, respectively.

One-year mortality following transplant has been associated with advanced donor age and recipient risk factors including extremes of age, prolonged allograft ischemic times (>200 min), significant renal failure requiring dialysis, and requirement for mechanical circulatory support [4]. For patients who survive beyond the first transplant year, mortality is predominantly related to immunosuppression. Risk factors for 5-year mortality include acute rejection, use of induction therapy (IL-2R antagonists), absence of cell-cycle inhibitors, calcineurin inhibitors, or mTOR inhibitors from the immunosuppression regimen, infection prior to transplant discharge, and dialysis requirements prior to transplant [4].

Primary causes of death within the first year of transplant include graft failure, infection, and acute rejection. Over time, mortality is predominantly driven by malignancy, graft failure, and the development of coronary allograft vasculopathy [4].

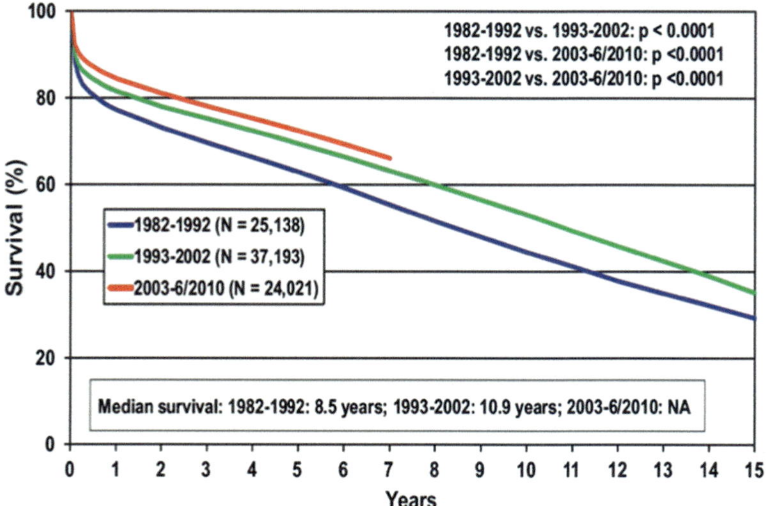

Fig. 6.1   Kaplan–Meier survival by era (adult heart transplants, January 1982 to June 2010) [4]

6.3.2   CF-LVAD

The survival benefit with mechanical circulatory support in patients with end-stage heart failure was first demonstrated in the seminal Randomized Evaluation of Mechanical Assistance for the Treatment of Congestive Heart Failure (REMATCH) trial [15]. This landmark study clearly showed a profound survival advantage for those who had been implanted with the pulsatile ventricular assist device. Specifically, 1- and 2-year survival rates on device support were 52 and 23 %, respectively, compared to the mortality rate of 75 and 92 % with optimal medical therapy.

However, pulsatile devices are rarely implanted in the current era having been replaced by the newer generation continuous-flow devices [16]. This was motivated by the results of the HeartMate II BTT and DT trials. Specifically, end-stage heart failure patients managed with CF-LVADs benefitted from a two-year actuarial survival of 58 % versus 24 % in the pulsatile device group in the HeartMate II DT trial [6]. Moreover, the complication profile significantly favored CF-LVADs including risk of device failure, strokes, bleeding, and infection. Similarly, CF-LVADs provided hemodynamic benefits for at least six months in patients awaiting cardiac transplantation [17].

More recently, the ADVANCE trial compared the HeartWare HVAD (Framingham, MA) to a contemporary INTERMACS control group [18]. The study findings were notable for a 90.7 % 6-month survival benefit in the HVAD group resulting in its FDA approval as a BTT CF-LVAD strategy. In addition, the study found that the contemporaneous CF-LVAD group had a similar survival rate of 90.1 % at 6 months. The original HeartMate II BTT trial demonstrated 1-year survival of 68 % [17], which improved to 85 % in the more recent data [19]. Other studies indicated that survival improvements have been at least sustained after wider spread of its use [16]. A post-FDA approval study for DT use of HeartMate II showed 2-year survival of 62 and 68 % for INTERMACS profile 4–7 versus 60 % for INTERMACS profile 1–3 [20]. In the INTERMACS Registry, 2-year survival of DT patients ($n = 1{,}694$) was approximately 60 %.

Mortality while on device support may arise from a multitude of causes arising from device-related complications and preexisting patient comorbidities. Specific etiologies leading to death include multi-organ failure, infection, bleeding, neurological events, and progression of underlying heart failure [16].

6.3.3   Cardiac Transplant Versus CF-LVAD

Comparing cardiac transplantation and CF-LVAD as heart replacement therapies is problematic owing to the paucity of head-to-head comparative data and the relative differences in patients eligible for either therapy.

Daneshmand et al. comparing their DT LVAD (pulsatile-flow LVAD) patients ($n = 60$) with patients who underwent high-risk cardiac transplantation ($n = 93$, the

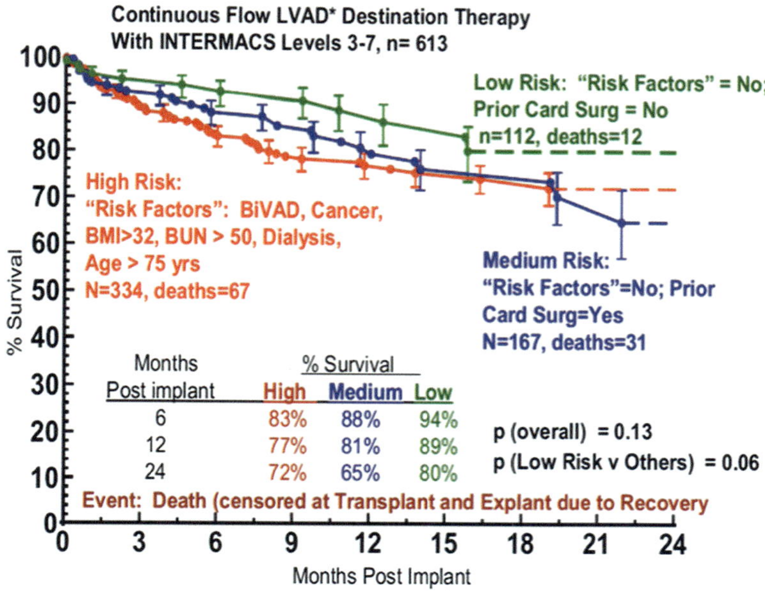

Months Post implant	% Survival		
	High	Medium	Low
6	83%	88%	94%
12	77%	81%	89%
24	72%	65%	80%

p (overall) = 0.13
p (Low Risk v Others) = 0.06

Fig. 6.2 Actuarial survival stratified by high-, medium-, and low-risk patients. "Risk factors" include presence of biventricular support, previous cancer, body mass index (BMI) greater than 32, serum sodium less than 130, or blood urea nitrogen (BUN) greater than 50 [24]. INTERMACS, Interagency Registry for Mechanically Assisted Circulatory Support; LVAD, left ventricular assist device

recipients in their extended criteria-alternate list who received a marginal donor heart) [21]. Thirty-day operative mortality and 1-year survival were 2.5 and 82 % for high-risk cardiac transplantation recipients and 6.7 and 77.5 % for DT LVAD patients (p=NS). Three-year survival was, however, better in high-risk cardiac transplantation patients (73 % vs. 50 % in DT LVAD).

The Columbia experience has also found essentially equivalent 1-year survival between DT LVAD, including both continuous and pulsatile devices, and transplant patients older than 65 years of age (83 % vs. 81 %, respectively) [22]. Other single-center experiences attest to similar one-year survival outcomes in patients with BTT CF-LVAD and cardiac transplant [23].

With a focus on LVAD therapy as a potential cardiac transplant replacement strategy, Kirklin et al. recently summarized a large body data from the INTERMACS Registry [24]. Between 2006 and 2011, 1,160 CF-LVADs were registered as a primary DT indication. CF-LVADs led to 1- and 2-year survival rates of 76 and 67 %, respectively. Further analysis of the DT cohort identified a subset of patients who were able to accomplish a transplant-comparable 2-year survival of 80 %. After the exclusion of those patients requiring biventricular support and notable preoperative risk factors, including cardiogenic shock, previous cancer, body mass index greater than 32 kg/m [2], serum sodium less than 130 mmol/L, blood urea nitrogen greater than 50 mg/dL, and previous cardiac surgery, DT patients within this cohort enjoyed 1- and 2-year survival rates of 88 % and 80 % after CF-LVAD implantation (Fig. 6.2).

Overall, approximately 20 % of their DT population experienced a 2-year survival equal to or greater than 80 %. This large registry data on DT patients, who in general have more comorbidities than those eligible for transplant, does seem to justify the concept of offering CF-LVAD to selected patients instead of cardiac transplantation in order to achieve equivalent survival outcomes at least in the midterm. However, it is too premature to be conclusive on the survival comparison between these two advanced therapies.

6.4 Adverse Events

6.4.1 Cardiac Transplantation

Acute rejection, coronary allograft vasculopathy (CAV), renal failure, and malignancy are amongst the most common morbidities that can lead to death in the cardiac transplant patient [4]. These morbidities are often closely linked to the consequences of immunosuppression and the immune interaction between the transplant recipient and the cardiac allograft. Though somewhat less frequent, rejection-related hospitalizations still occur at a rate of 22 % within 1 year and 36 % within 3 years of transplantation [4]. CAV develops in approximately 10 % of recipients within 1 year and more than half by 10 years. The development of CAV is closely linked to both graft failure and ultimate patient death. Survival has improved owing to newer approaches to the treatment of CAV, including the use of statins to lower LDL-cholesterol levels and the addition of mTOR inhibitors to the immunosuppressive regimen. Revascularization with drug-eluting coronary stents has been studied but with variable results. The incidence of renal failure, typically the consequence of calcineurin inhibitor use, is approximately 6 % at 1 year and 16 % at 5 years. Malignancy arises as later complication following transplant with an incidence of non-skin cancer of 1 % at 1 year, 6 % at 5 years, 15 % at 10 years, and 24 % at 15 years. Opportunistic infections may also increase hospital readmissions and the potential risk for death. We have observed an 11 % incidence of pneumonia within the first year after cardiac transplant which was associated with 1-year survival reduction by 9 % [25]. Other non-life-threatening, yet significant post-transplant complications, may further affect a patient's quality of life. Cardiovascular side effects including hypertension, diabetes mellitus and dyslipidemia, or cosmetic changes resulting from long-standing corticosteroid use have a substantial impact on patients' quality of life.

6.4.2 CF-LVAD

With the introduction of CF-LVADs, the adverse event profile that significantly complicated the durability of the early generation pulsatile devices has significantly improved. However, the incidence and their clinical significance of such complications remain nontrivial. The reported adverse event rates per 100 patient months are 1.6 for device malfunction, 9.45 for bleeding events, 1.79 in right ventricular failure, 4.66 in cardiac arrhythmia, 8.01 for infection, 1.83 for neurological events, and 1.83 in renal dysfunction in the first year after CF-LVAD implantation [16]. We have reported a 10 % or 0.16 events per patient year incidence of cerebrovascular accidents, including hemorrhagic or ischemic strokes, with the HeartMate II CF-LVAD [26]. Large registry data have demonstrated a nearly 19 % incidence of driveline infection in CF-LVAD recipients at 1 year after CF-LVAD implantation [27].

In addition to these adverse events, longer-term mechanical support has further revealed undesired complications arising from non-pulsatile continuous flow. CF-LVAD use is almost inevitably associated with the development of an acquired von Willebrand syndrome, which, when coupled with obligate device anticoagulation, contributes to high incidence of bleeding events [28]. In addition, nearly 25 % of patients develop de novo aortic insufficiency within the first year following CF-LVAD implantation [29]. In our experience, freedom from moderate or greater aortic insufficiency was 88 and 65 % at 1 and 2 years, respectively. Patients with consequent refractory symptoms or heart failure from device-related aortic insufficiency often require surgical intervention including aortic valve repair or urgent cardiac transplantation [30].

6.4.3 Cardiac Transplantation Versus CF-LVAD

Cardiac transplantation and CF-LVAD therapy have unique and specific complication profiles associated with their use and render head-to-head comparisons challenging. As such, it is difficult to conclude which therapy is "better" from an adverse event profile. Understandably, choice between device and transplant requires a thorough evaluation of underlying patient comorbidity, eligibility for transplant, and ultimately, patient preference.

6.5 Quality of Life

Both cardiac transplant and CF-LVAD therapies result in a remarkable improvement in survival in appropriately selected patients with stage D heart failure. Of equal importance to survival is the restoration and preservation of quality of life and the facility of an active lifestyle after either strategy. Accordingly, nearly 90 % of patients in the first 5 years after transplant have no significant limitations to activity. Approximately 50 % of patients who were transplanted between the ages of 25 and 55 years are employed at 3 years following their transplant [19]. In contrast, quality of life data are somewhat limited in patients on mechanical circulatory support. Available data suggest an important and sustained improvement in general well-being, self-care, and performance of usual activities within the first year following device implantation [16]. However, many patients continue to experience at least some level of emotional distress with their device related to uncertainty, fear of device failure, and anxiety. A review of self-reported patient outcomes found that despite an improvement in overall clinical status beyond the first 3 months after either pulsatile or continuous-flow device implantation, LVAD patients experienced considerably poorer physical and mental health and social functioning both at baseline and 6 months in follow-up as compared to transplant recipients [31].

6.6   Cost

The cost of heart failure management places a huge burden on health-care resources and accounts for 2 % to 5 % of the total health-care budget in most developed countries [32,33]. The expenditure associated with heart transplant and LVAD therapy is in excess of that required in the treatment of various advanced stage medical illnesses [34]. However, the true cost of cardiac transplantation may be underestimated and never be fully realized due to the limited donor heart supply that does not meet the overall heart failure patient population need.

Cost-effectiveness of advanced heart failure management may be further evaluated using economic metrics such quality of adjusted life year (QALY), which takes into account both survival benefit and improvement in quality of life with a medical intervention. It has been suggested that a cost-effectiveness ratio of less than $20,000 per QALY to be very attractive; a ratio of $20,000 to $60,000 per QALY acceptable; a ratio of $60,000 to $100,000 per QALY is less than desirable; and a ratio greater than $100,000 per QALY to be unattractive [35]. As such, the incremental cost-effectiveness ratio of LVADs would need to be at a minimum less than $100,000 per QALY to be considered to be reasonably cost-effective, albeit still more expensive than would be desired. Based on analyses from the HeartMate II Destination Therapy trial, the cost-effectiveness of CF-LVAD therapy was $198,184 per QALY and $167,208 per life year [36]. Even after appreciating that well-conducted cost-effectiveness studies may be limited by many layers of uncertainty in measuring efficacy and economic data, it is clear that LVAD therapy is *extremely expensive*. Although it is an off-the-shelf treatment modality, its unregulated use may result in an unsustainable economic burden to both patient and society. As such, LVAD therapy, much like the donor heart pool, is also a limited resource, particularly if mechanical support therapy is to be used judiciously in the face of such economic constraints. However, the cost-effectiveness of LVAD therapy will inevitably be dynamic with the evolution of device technology and cumulative clinical experience. As such, modifications to survival and readmission metrics resulting from improved patient selection and overall device management will ultimately impact economic calculations. In fact a significant decrease in cost was demonstrated in patients with HeartMate II CF-LVADs as compared to the early generation pulsatile HeartMate I device after targeted efforts focused on reducing device costs, time in critical care units, and overall hospital lengths of stay resulting from readmissions from complications.

6.7 Functional Recovery of the Native Heart

In some patients, LVAD support facilitates sufficient myocardial recovery of left ventricular function to permit device explantation. In a retrospective analysis of more than one thousand clinical trial patients with HeartMate II LVADs, the overall device explantation rate due to myocardial recovery was 1.8 % [37].

LVAD therapy may also offer the opportunity in combination with other types of strategies to promote significant improvement in the structure and function of the failing myocardium [38]. The Harefield protocol consists of a combined approach of LVAD therapy with aggressive pharmacological neurohormonal blockade (phase I). Phase II of this protocol entails the introduction of clenbuterol, a sympathomimetic amine with $\beta2$ agonist properties known to promote physiologic myocardial hypertrophy, to the pharmacological regimen. With this protocol, myocardial recovery was observed in approximately two thirds of patients with a non-ischemic cardiomyopathy [39]. This experience prompted the Harefield Recovery Protocol Study (HARPS), which failed to replicate the result. However, the strategy of combining pharmacological therapy with mechanical unloading to promote myocardial recovery continues to be an appealing therapeutic intervention [40,41].

Another strategy on the therapeutic horizon is the potential role of regenerative medicine in the treatment of end-stage heart disease. Enormous strides have been achieved over the last 10 years, highlighted by promising clinical trial results emerging from stem cell strategies aimed at treating myocardial infarction [42,43]. The coincidental evolution of LVAD therapy and the field of regeneration medicine has opened a window for novel therapeutic approaches to advanced heart failure management [44]. In fact, a multicenter study in which patients were randomized to receive stem cell injections within the myocardium at the time of LVAD implantation has just finished enrolment. Such interventions to promote recovery of native heart function are not feasible with cardiac transplantation.

6.8 Conclusions

Mechanical circulatory support devices will continue to "challenge" the role of cardiac transplantation as the definitive heart replacement strategy in patients with end-stage heart failure. Two major reasons for this challenge are related to "device availability" and anticipated "technological advances" that will lead to improve clinical outcomes with device therapy. There is no doubt that CF-LVADs are more readily available than donor hearts. In fact, CF-LVADs are now an off-the-shelf treatment modality for eligible patients. One caveat, however, is the relative prohibitive cost associated with device therapy, which may limit its greater penetration within the heart failure population.

The success of mechanical circulatory support has predominantly been derived from technological advancements, highlighted by the development of the rotary flow pump. Ultimately, innovative engineering will drive the evolution of the next generation of pumps, their expansion to biventricular support, and the development

Table 6.1 Comparison between cardiac transplantation and CF-LVAD

Factors	Cardiac transplantation	CF-LVAD
Survival		
1 year (%)	90	70–90
2 years (%)	80	60–80
5 years (%)	70	Unknown
10 years (%)	50	Unknown
Adverse events	Rejection, CAV, renal failure, malignancy, infection, diabetes mellitus, cosmetic side effects	RV failure, bleeding, CVA, infection, renal dysfunction, device malfunction, AI
Quality of life	Good	Somewhat limited
Availability	Limited	Good
Cost		
Per patient	Expensive	Expensive
To society	Not too expensive due to limited donor availability	Could become very expensive if volume expands
Myocardial recovery	Not feasible	Feasible
Future advance	Maybe	Definitely

AI aortic insufficiency, *CAV* cardiac allograft vasculopathy, *CF-LVAD* continuous-flow left ventricular assist device, *CVA* cerebrovascular accident, *RV* right ventricular

of transcutaneous energy transmission systems that will render the infection prone driveline nonexistent. As such, the expansion of device-based therapy in both clinical indication and numbers of patients who may benefit from improved survival and quality of life holds great promise. Moreover, the complementary use of such novel device strategies with new pharmacological therapies and/or regenerative medicine offers the potential for myocardial recovery. In contrast, despite its place as the "gold standard" treatment for refractory heart failure, progress in cardiac transplantation science has remained relatively static.

An overall comparison of cardiac transplantation and CF-LVAD therapy is summarized in Table 6.1. In this era, current evidence indicates that cardiac transplantation is a good and reliable therapy supported by a strong and historic record of clinical success. In contrast, mechanical circulatory support devices, currently represented by CF-LVADs, provide a reasonable midterm clinical outcome in patients with end-stage heart failure. The promising future of mechanical circulatory support will be further realized as the cumulative clinical experience with device therapy grows.

Importantly, neither cardiac transplantation nor CF-LVAD therapy is curative for end-stage heart disease. Both provide a relative finite extension of life expectancy that is encumbered by a long list of complications unique to each strategy. More data, especially longer follow-up with CF-LVAD therapy, and ideally a head-to-head comparison of both therapies will be required to answer the question: *can CF-LVAD therapy replace cardiac transplantation as the preferred treatment for advanced heart disease?* In the current era, however, it is most essential that the complementary nature of both therapies be appreciated, along with a clear understanding of the differences in their indications, benefits, and complication profiles to ensure the best achievable outcome for the patient with end-stage heart failure.

References

1. Hunt SA, Abraham WT, Chin MH, Feldman AM, Francis GS, Ganiats TG, et al. American College of Cardiology F, American Heart A. 2009 focused update incorporated into the acc/aha 2005 guidelines for the diagnosis and management of heart failure in adults a report of the american college of cardiology foundation/american heart association task force on practice guidelines developed in collaboration with the international society for heart and lung transplantation. J Am Coll Cardiol. 2009;53:e1–90.
2. Stevenson LW, Kormos RL, Bourge RC, Gelijns A, Griffith BP, Hershberger RE, et al. Mechanical cardiac support 2000: current applications and future trial design. June 15–16, 2000 Bethesda, Maryland. J Am Coll Cardiol. 2001;37:340–70.
3. Garbade J, Barten MJ, Bittner HB, Mohr FW. Heart transplantation and left ventricular assist device therapy: two comparable options in end-stage heart failure? Clin Cardiol. 2013;36(7):378–82.
4. Stehlik J, Edwards LB, Kucheryavaya AY, Benden C, Christie JD, Dipchand AI, et al. International Society of H, Lung T. The registry of the international society for heart and lung transplantation: 29th official adult heart transplant report–2012. J Heart Lung Transplant. 2012;31:1052–64.
5. U.S. Department of Health and Human Services. Heathcare Systems Bureau, Division of Transplantation, Editor. Rockville: ARotUSOPaTNatSRoTRTD-HRaSA; 2009.
6. Slaughter MS, Rogers JG, Milano CA, Russell SD, Conte JV, Feldman D, et al. Advanced heart failure treated with continuous-flow left ventricular assist device. N Engl J Med. 2009;361:2241–51.
7. Kormos RL, Teuteberg JJ, Pagani FD, Russell SD, John R, Miller LW, et al. Right ventricular failure in patients with the heartmate II continuous-flow left ventricular assist device: incidence, risk factors, and effect on outcomes. J Thorac Cardiovasc Surg. 2010;139:1316–24.
8. Matthews JC, Koelling TM, Pagani FD, Aaronson KD. The right ventricular failure risk score a pre-operative tool for assessing the risk of right ventricular failure in left ventricular assist device candidates. J Am Coll Cardiol. 2008;51:2163–72.
9. Fitzpatrick 3rd JR, Frederick JR, Hsu VM, Kozin ED, O'Hara ML, Howell E, et al. Risk score derived from pre-operative data analysis predicts the need for biventricular mechanical circulatory support. J Heart Lung Transplant. 2008;27:1286–92.
10. Grant AD, Smedira NG, Starling RC, Marwick TH. Independent and incremental role of quantitative right ventricular evaluation for the prediction of right ventricular failure after left ventricular assist device implantation. J Am Coll Cardiol. 2012;60:521–8.
11. Goda A, Takayama H, Koeckert M, Pak SW, Sutton EM, Cohen S, et al. Use of ventricular assist devices in patients with mitral valve prostheses. J Cardiac Surg. 2011;26:334–7.
12. Goda A, Takayama H, Pak SW, Uriel N, Mancini D, Naka Y, et al. Aortic valve procedures at the time of ventricular assist device placement. Ann Thorac Surg. 2011;91:750–4.
13. Mikus E, Stepanenko A, Krabatsch T, Loforte A, Dandel M, Lehmkuhl HB, et al. Reversibility of fixed pulmonary hypertension in left ventricular assist device support recipients. Eur J Cardiothorac Surg. 2011;40:971–7.
14. Everly MJ. Cardiac transplantation in the united states: an analysis of the unos registry. Clin Transpl. 2008;35–43.
15. Rose EA, Gelijns AC, Moskowitz AJ, Heitjan DF, Stevenson LW, Dembitsky W, et al. Randomized evaluation of mechanical assistance for the treatment of congestive heart failure study G. Long-term use of a left ventricular assist device for end-stage heart failure. N Engl J Med. 2001;345:1435–43.
16. Kirklin JK, Naftel DC, Kormos RL, Stevenson LW, Pagani FD, Miller MA, et al. Fifth intermacs annual report: Risk factor analysis from more than 6,000 mechanical circulatory support patients. J Heart Lung Transplant. 2013;32:141–56.

17. Miller LW, Pagani FD, Russell SD, John R, Boyle AJ, Aaronson KD, et al. Use of a continuous-flow device in patients awaiting heart transplantation. N Engl J Med. 2007;357:885–96.

18. Aaronson KD, Slaughter MS, Miller LW, McGee EC, Cotts WG, Acker MA, et al. HeartWare Ventricular Assist Device Bridge to Transplant ATI. Use of an intrapericardial, continuous-flow, centrifugal pump in patients awaiting heart transplantation. Circulation. 2012;125:3191–200.

19. Starling RC, Naka Y, Boyle AJ, Gonzalez-Stawinski G, John R, Jorde U, et al. Results of the post-U.S. food and drug administration-approval study with a continuous flow left ventricular assist device as a bridge to heart transplantation: a prospective study using the intermacs (interagency registry for mechanically assisted circulatory support). J Am Coll Cardiol. 2011;57:1890–8.

20. Jorde U, Khushwaha AJ, Tatooles AJ, Naka Y, Bhat G, Long JW, et al. Two-year outcomes in the destination therapy post-fda-approval study with a continuous flow left ventricular assist device: a prospective study using the intermacs registry. J Heart Lung Transplant. 2013;32:S10.

21. Daneshmand MA, Rajagopal K, Lima B, Khorram N, Blue LJ, Lodge AJ, et al. Left ventricular assist device destination therapy versus extended criteria cardiac transplant. Ann Thorac Surg. 2010;89:1205–9. discussion 1210.

22. Melnitchouk S, Jorde U, Takayama H, Uriel N, Colombo PC, Yang J, et al. Continuous-flow lvad destination therapy versus orthotopic heart transplantation in patients above 65 years of age. J Heart Lung Transplant. 2011;30:S94–5.

23. Williams ML, Trivedi JR, McCants KC, Prabhu SD, Birks EJ, Oliver L, et al. Heart transplant vs left ventricular assist device in heart transplant-eligible patients. Ann thorac Surg. 2011;91:1330–3. discussion 1333–1334.

24. Kirklin JK, Naftel DC, Pagani FD, Kormos RL, Stevenson L, Miller M, et al. Long-term mechanical circulatory support (destination therapy): on track to compete with heart transplantation? J Thorac Cardiovasc Surg. 2012;144:584–603. discussion 597–588.

25. Uriel N, Pak SW, Hayashi Y, Gukasayan N, Tsiouris SJ, Scully BE, et al. Pneumonia in the first year after heart transplant: Epidemiology, risk factors, and effect on survival. J Cardiac Fail. 2010;16:S55.

26. Kato TS, Schulze PC, Yang J, Chan E, Shahzad K, Takayama H, et al. Pre-operative and post-operative risk factors associated with neurologic complications in patients with advanced heart failure supported by a left ventricular assist device. J Heart Lung Transplant. 2012;31:1–8.

27. Goldstein DJ, Naftel D, Holman W, Bellumkonda L, Pamboukian SV, Pagani FD, et al. Continuous-flow devices and percutaneous site infections: clinical outcomes. J Heart Lung Transplant. 2012;31:1151–7.

28. Uriel N, Pak SW, Jorde UP, Jude B, Susen S, Vincentelli A, et al. Acquired von willebrand syndrome after continuous-flow mechanical device support contributes to a high prevalence of bleeding during long-term support and at the time of transplantation. J Am Coll Cardiol. 2010;56:1207–13.

29. Pak SW, Uriel N, Takayama H, Cappleman S, Song R, Colombo PC, et al. Prevalence of de novo aortic insufficiency during long-term support with left ventricular assist devices. J Heart lung Transplant. 2010;29:1172–6.

30. Bejar D, Nahumi N, Uriel N, Thomas S, Han J, Garan A, et al. The prevalence of aortic insufficiency in patients maintained on continuous flow left ventricular assist devices. J Heart Lung Transplant. 2013;32:S185.

31. Brouwers C, Denollet J, de Jonge N, Caliskan K, Kealy J, Pedersen SS. Patient-reported outcomes in left ventricular assist device therapy: a systematic review and recommendations for clinical research and practice. Circ Heart Fail. 2011;4:714–23.

32. Cowie MR, Cure S, Bianic F, McGuire A, Goodall G, Tavazzi L. Cost-effectiveness of highly purified omega-3 polyunsaturated fatty acid ethyl esters in the treatment of chronic heart failure: Results of markov modelling in a uk setting. Eur J Heart Fail. 2011;13:681–9.

33. Heidenreich PA, Trogdon JG, Khavjou OA, Butler J, Dracup K, Ezekowitz MD, et al. American Heart Association Advocacy Coordinating C, Stroke C, Council on Cardiovascular R, Intervention, Council on Clinical C, Council on E, Prevention, Council on A, Thrombosis,

Vascular B, Council on C, Critical C, Perioperative, Resuscitation, Council on Cardiovascular N, Council on the Kidney in Cardiovascular D, Council on Cardiovascular S, Anesthesia, Interdisciplinary Council on Quality of C Outcomes R. Forecasting the future of cardiovascular disease in the united states: A policy statement from the american heart association. Circulation. 2011;123:933–44.

34. Miller LW, Guglin M, Rogers J. Cost of ventricular assist devices: can we afford the progress? Circulation. 2013;127:743–8.

35. Goldman L, Gordon DJ, Rifkind BM, Hulley SB, Detsky AS, Goodman DW, et al. Cost and health implications of cholesterol lowering. Circulation. 1992;85:1960–8.

36. Rogers JG, Bostic RR, Tong KB, Adamson R, Russo M, Slaughter MS. Cost-effectiveness analysis of continuous-flow left ventricular assist devices as destination therapy. Circ Heart Fail. 2012;5:10–6.

37. Goldstein DJ, Maybaum S, MacGillivray TE, Moore SA, Bogaev R, Farrar DJ, et al. Young patients with nonischemic cardiomyopathy have higher likelihood of left ventricular recovery during left ventricular assist device support. J Cardiac Fail. 2012;18:392–5.

38. Ibrahim M, Terracciano C, Yacoub MH. Can bridge to recovery help to reveal the secrets of the failing heart? Curr Cardiol Rep. 2012;14:392–6.

39. Birks EJ, Tansley PD, Hardy J, George RS, Bowles CT, Burke M, et al. Left ventricular assist device and drug therapy for the reversal of heart failure. N Engl J Med. 2006;355:1873–84.

40. Birks EJ, George RS, Hedger M, Bahrami T, Wilton P, Bowles CT, et al. Reversal of severe heart failure with a continuous-flow left ventricular assist device and pharmacological therapy: a prospective study. Circulation. 2011;123:381–90.

41. Patel SR, Saeed O, Murthy S, Bhatia V, Shin JJ, Wang D, et al. Combining neurohormonal blockade with continuous-flow left ventricular assist device support for myocardial recovery: a single-arm prospective study. J Heart Lung Transplant. 2013;32:305–12.

42. Hou J, Wang L, Jiang J, Zhou C, Guo T, Zheng S, et al. Cardiac stem cells and their roles in myocardial infarction. Stem Cell Rev. 2013;9(3):326–38.

43. Chugh AR, Beache GM, Loughran JH, Mewton N, Elmore JB, Kajstura J, et al. Administration of cardiac stem cells in patients with ischemic cardiomyopathy: the scipio trial: Surgical aspects and interim analysis of myocardial function and viability by magnetic resonance. Circulation. 2012;126:S54–64.

44. Ibrahim M, Rao C, Athanasiou T, Yacoub MH, Terracciano CM. Mechanical unloading and cell therapy have a synergistic role in the recovery and regeneration of the failing heart. Eur J Cardiothorac Surg. 2012;42:312–8.

Chapter 7
Strategies to Assess and Minimize Right Heart Failure After Left Ventricular Assist Device Implantation

Michihito Nonaka and Vivek Rao

Abstract *Objective*: Despite the positive effects of decreased right ventricular afterload after implantation of a left ventricular assist device, the right ventricle may also sustain negative effects through changes in position of the interventricular septum and perioperative tricuspid regurgitation. Right ventricular failure, which occurs in 20–50 % of patients after left ventricular assist device implantation, is associated with substantial operative mortality and morbidity. *Methods*: This article reviews the pathology of and risk factors and management strategies for right ventricle failure after left ventricular assist device implantation. *Results*: Risk factors are female gender, non-ischemic cardiomyopathy, and preoperative mechanical support or intra-aortic balloon pumping; however, the significance of these findings was limited. Risk scoring systems have been developed to quantify this risk. Inotropes that induce pulmonary vasodilation, e.g., milrinone, accompanied by inotropes that increase systolic blood pressure, i.e., epinephrine, for coronary perfusion, are effective treatments for right ventricular failure. A specific pulmonary vasodilator, such as inhaled nitric oxide, which reduces pulmonary vascular resistance and increases device flow, is another important component of therapy. Because valvular pathologies can complicate postoperative management, correction of tricuspid regurgitation is necessary to decrease venous congestion and improve right ventricle function. *Conclusions*: Meticulous attention should be paid to optimizing preload, afterload, and contractility in patients with preexisting right ventricular dysfunction in order to prevent right ventricle failure after left ventricular assist device implantation. For intraoperative right ventricle failure, alternative measures of mechanical support, including a right ventricular assist device as a last resort, are used.

Keywords Assessment • Left ventricular assist device • Right heart failure • Treatment

M. Nonaka • V. Rao (⊠)
Department of Cardiovascular Surgery, Toronto General Hospital, Toronto, ON, Canada
e-mail: Vivek.Rao@uhn.ca

S. Kyo (ed.), *Ventricular Assist Devices in Advanced-Stage Heart Failure*,
DOI 10.1007/978-4-431-54466-1_7, © Springer Japan 2014

7.1 Introduction

Insertion of a ventricular assist device (VAD) has become an established procedure for patients with end-stage heart failure, with acceptable outcomes for either destination therapy (DT) or bridge-to-transplant (BTT) indications. With technological advancement, non-pulsatile flow devices have produced superior outcomes compared to the earlier pulsatile devices [1–3].

Right ventricular (RV) dysfunction is one of the most critical complications after left ventricular assist device (LVAD) implantation. Some studies have reported that the incidence of post-LVAD implantation RV failure is between 20 % and 50 % [1–5] and that this failure rate has not decreased significantly despite the advances in LVAD technology [6, 7]. RV failure after LVAD implantation is associated with higher operative mortality and morbidity and longer stays in intensive care units and hospitals [8, 9]. The development of RV failure after LVAD implantation reduces survival even after heart transplantation [10]. Therefore, it is important to diagnose and appropriately treat RV failure in LVAD patients. This article reviews the pathology of RV failure and management strategies for RV failure after LVAD implantation.

7.2 Physiology of the Right Ventricle

7.2.1 Normal Right Ventricle

The structure and mechanical function of the RV differs from that of the left ventricle (LV), and the RV responds differently to disease. Anatomically, the RV is a complex three-dimensional structure located in the anterior part of the heart beneath the sternum [11]. It has a triangular configuration in sagittal section and is crescent shaped in cross section, with the interventricular septum (IVS) concave towards the LV. The shape and function of the RV are influenced by the projection of the IVS, which is an important factor in abnormal loading status. The RV and the LV have a significant correlation to input and output of systemic volume.

Contraction of the RV through its highly compliant thin wall starts at the inlet ending at the infundibulum (the RV outflow tract). The RV sends blood to the highly compliant pulmonary system, which functions as a volume pump with low pressure rather than as a pressure pump. Through the cardiac cycle, the RV generates a stroke volume equal to the LV stroke volume, with 25 % of the stroke work [12]. Because the RV has a greater end-diastolic volume than that of the LV, the ejection fraction (EF) of the RV is less (RVEF, 40–45 %) than that of the LV (LVEF, 50–55 %) [13]. Increased pulmonary artery pressure (PAP) is associated with decreased RVEF. Because the RV is more sensitive to afterload change than the LV, the same increase in afterload causes a greater decrease in the stroke volume of the RV compared to the LV [14]. On the other hand, the RV adapts more easily to volume overload.

The RV receives coronary perfusion during both systolic and diastolic phases of the cardiac cycle. Lower stroke work and wall stress leads to lower resting coronary flow (0.4–0.7 mL min^{-1} g^{-1} myocardium) and oxygen extraction (50 % vs. 75 %) for the RV vs. LV [15]. With these flow and oxygen extraction reserves, the RV is more resilient to ischemia.

The two ventricles have significant interdependence, in which the shape, size, and compliance of one ventricle affects those of the other through direct mechanical interactions [11, 14]. This interdependence is regulated by the IVS in the systolic phase and by the pericardium in the diastolic phase. Ventricular interdependence is an important factor in the loading conditions for both ventricles.

7.2.2 Right Ventricular Failure

The causes of RV failure can be classified as intrinsic RV failure without pulmonary hypertension, i.e., RV infarction; RV failure due to increased RV afterload; and RV failure caused by volume overload [15].

Pulmonary hypertension is a common condition in both systolic and diastolic left heart failure. RV failure due to increased afterload occurs through a series of physiological steps. First, in the systolic phase, the increased afterload delays the timing of the opening of the pulmonary valve, which prolongs isovolumic contraction time. Isovolumic contraction consumes more oxygen because it involves pressure work rather than volume work. In the next phase, the compliant RV dilates to maintain stroke volume by the Frank–Starling mechanism. However, as dictated by the Law of Laplace, this dilatation of the RV causes an increase in myocardial wall stress. The increased myocardial stress also increases oxygen demand. At the same time, elevated RV end-diastolic pressure leads to deterioration of right coronary perfusion. Thus, the oxygen supply to the RV myocardium decreases, further disrupting the balance between the supply and demand of oxygen.

Dilation of the RV cavity causes dilatation of the tricuspid annulus, resulting in tricuspid regurgitation (TR), which further exacerbates the dilatation of RV. Over time, increased wall stress leads to hypertrophy of the RV muscle. As the RV expands, the shape of the RV chamber is distorted, and eventually the IVS will be pushed further to the LV side. Because the pericardium limits the space of the heart, increased RV volume will be compensated by a decreased LV volume. Septal bulging to the LV side affects filling of the LV chamber and therefore impairs LV function. With impaired LV function, coronary perfusion will decrease, further deteriorating RV function.

In cases of severe RV failure, high venous pressure accompanied with reduced systemic pressure affects perfusion of the major organs, as is manifested by signs such as decrease in urine output due to renal hypoperfusion and coagulation abnormalities and elevated liver enzymes due to hepatic hypoperfusion. Without appropriate treatment for RV overloading, a vicious cycle is established and may eventually lead to circulatory collapse, multiple-organ failure, and death.

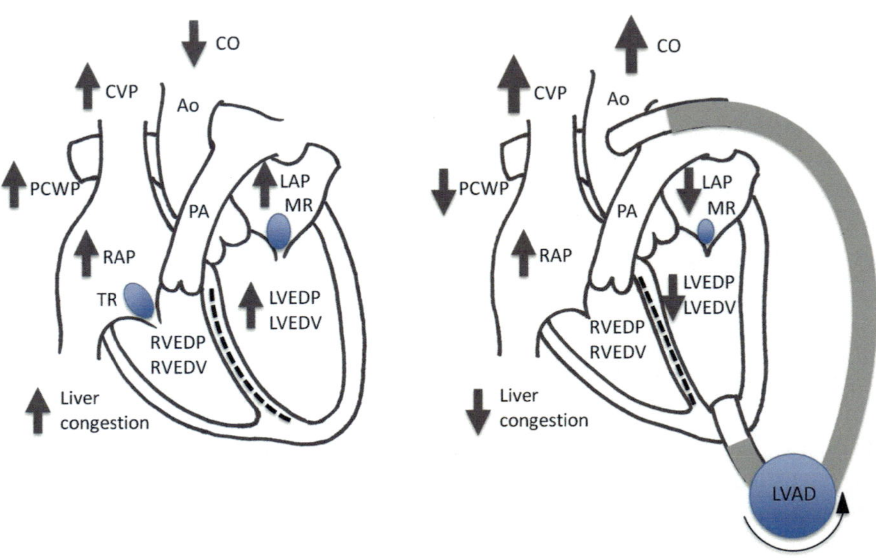

Fig. 7.1 Heart failure and LVAD physiology. *Ao* aorta, *PA* pulmonary artery, *LVAD* left ventricular assist device, *MR* mitral regurgitation, *TR* tricuspid regurgitation, *CO* cardiac output, *CVP* central venous pressure, *LAP* left atrial pressure, *PCWP* pulmonary capillary wedge pressure, *RAP* right atrial pressure, *LVEDP* left ventricular end-diastolic pressure, *LVEDV* left ventricular end-diastolic volume, *RVEDP* right ventricular end-diastolic pressure, *RVEDV* right ventricular end-diastolic volume

RV failure can occur under conditions of normal RV afterload, as in the case of RV myocardial infarction (MI). RV MI is caused by disease in the right coronary artery or dominant left circumflex artery. Although isolated RV infarction may have been overlooked compared to LV infarction, the significance of the high mortality associated with isolated RV infarction has recently become more clear [16].

7.2.3 Right Ventricular Failure After Left Ventricular Assist Device Implantation

RV function is influenced positively and negatively by LVAD (Fig. 7.1). Sufficient LVAD circulation requires the RV to increase its output in order to match the LVAD flow. Augmentation of systemic flow by the LVAD also increases venous return to the RV. Diastolic compliance of the RV improves in response to the increased pre-load, accompanied by decreased RV afterload and a leftward shift of the IVS because the LVAD reduces LV pressure. RV function is maintained as long as the unloaded RV does not need to contract harder to eject the increased RV preload [6, 17–19], and in the clinical setting, this is manifested as a decrease in pulmonary capillary wedge pressure (PCWP), PAP, and peak RV systolic pressure (RVSP).

Despite the positive effects of decreased RV afterload, the RV may also sustain negative effects influenced by the LVAD. RV function is related to contraction of its free wall and the position of the IVS. During LVAD support, RV contractility may be impaired by changes in IVS position and motion. When the LV is excessively unloaded, the IVS shifts markedly towards the LV and impairs efficient RV contraction. To compensate for the loss of IVS function, the workload of the free wall of the RV increases, causing exhaustion of the RV.

LVAD implantation causes an inconsistent change in the extent of perioperative TR. The severity of TR is worsened by the leftward shift of the IVS as well as increased pulmonary vascular resistance (PVR) caused by cardiopulmonary bypass (CPB), systemic inflammatory response syndrome (SIRS), and increased preload after blood transfusion. In addition, high flow of the LVAD may distort the tricuspid valve annulus.

7.3 Definition of Right Ventricular Failure

The preoperative condition of patients who require LVAD implantation includes a broad presentation of RV dysfunction, from asymptomatic to severe RV failure (RVF). In this patient population, RVF is defined as a clinical syndrome characterized by decreased ability of the RV to fill and eject appropriately or impaired function of the RV in providing adequate blood flow through the pulmonary circulation at a normal preload [20].

There has been no universal definition of RVF after LVAD implantation among authors because of the retrospective nature of the available studies. RVF occurs when the pulmonary circulation is unable to fill the LVAD despite maximal medical therapy. The need for a right ventricular assist device (RVAD) is accepted as an indicator of extreme RVF, and even without requiring RVAD, RVF is considered when conditions are such that hemodynamic instability requires pharmacological support, i.e., inotropes or pulmonary vasodilators, for >2 weeks. Patients with RV failure may also require a combination of the two [4, 6, 8, 21–23].

Potapov et al. have developed specific hemodynamic and inotropic support criteria as indicators for introduction of inhaled nitric oxide (*i*NO) therapy to manage RVF [24], and Hennig et al. used similar hemodynamic definitions of RVF as indicators for *i*NO treatment [7].

7.4 Evaluation of Right Ventricular Function

7.4.1 Modalities to Evaluate Right Ventricular Function

Right heart assessment is important for monitoring RV function and identifying possible causes of RV dysfunction. Assessment of the RV is sometimes challenging because of its anterior retrosternal position, complex geometry, and hemodynamic load dependence.

Echocardiography has been the most common method for RV evaluation. Three-dimensional echocardiography is a promising modality that can provide more accurate evaluation, although cardiac magnetic resonance imaging (MRI) has become a standard. Assessment of RV structure should include observations of the RV size, shape, volume, and wall thickness [25], and MRI is now considered the most reliable method for measuring RV volume [26, 27]. RVEF and RV fractional area change (RVFAC) are calculated on the basis of size and volume measurements determined by the imaging studies.

Tricuspid valve (TV) annular plane systolic excursion (TAPSE), which is an echocardiographic measurement of the longitudinal displacement of the TV annulus during systole, is used for evaluation of RV function. Displacement >15 mm in TAPSE is a quantitative measure of normal RV systolic function. However, TAPSE is less reliable in patients with focal RV dysfunction because it only measures the longitudinal movement of the lateral free wall. Evaluation of the TV annulus size, the presence and severity of TR, the inferior vena cava size, and the hepatic venous blood flow pattern are also important parts of the evaluation of RV function. Although there is good correlation among TAPSE, RVFAC, and RVEF, many cardiographers use a subjective assessment that classifies global RV function as good or as mildly, moderately, or severely reduced.

7.4.2 Evaluation After Left Ventricular Assist Device Implantation

Echocardiography is the primary imaging modality for evaluating cardiac function after LVAD implantation because MRI is not an option for patients with these devices [27]. Changes in RV size and the degree of TR are followed serially. When RV function is worsening, RV size and the extent of TR increase correspondingly.

In patients with LVAD, a decrease in the TAPSE is seen because RV afterload and RV contractile work to maintain cardiac output (CO) are reduced [17]. However, low TAPSE in the presence of increasing RV size and TR suggests worsening RV function [28].

An important structural feature in evaluation of heart function is the position the IVS, as it reflects various factors. A shift of the IVS may indicate RV dysfunction, inappropriate volume loading, incorrect LVAD setting, and LVAD device failure. Because of the space limitations imposed by the pericardium, potential right heart compression by fluid collection or thrombus should also be considered.

With continuous-flow LVAD support, preexisting RV dysfunction was not exacerbated during a median follow-up of 4.5 months [29]. Moreover, the size of RV chamber is reduced in parallel with that of the LV chamber, although the degree of the change in the RV is variable. In contrast, the pulsatile LVADs consistently decompressed the LV to a greater degree, thus impairing RV function by leftward shifting of the IVS.

7.5 Predictors of RV Failure

7.5.1 Risk Factors

Many studies have attempted to identify preoperative risk factors and develop risk scores in order to identify patients at the greatest risk for postoperative RV failure after LVAD implantation and to formulate the appropriate treatment strategies for them. Patients at high risk for postoperative RV failure would receive benefits from preoperative optimization of RV function and possibly even planned biventricular assist device (BiVAD) support. However, it is still difficult to predict the incidence of postoperative RV failure in the LVAD patients because RV failure includes multiple factors throughout the treatment.

Some studies have identified particular patient characteristics and hemodynamic parameters as risk factors for postoperative RV failure, but the significance of the findings is limited by small cohorts, single institution, retrospective nature, and inconsistent use of an LVAD type.

According to published studies, preoperative risk factors for postoperative RV failure in patients with LVAD are female gender; non-ischemic cardiomyopathy [30]; preoperative support, including mechanical ventilation, mechanical circulatory support [4, 8, 23], or intra-aortic balloon pumping (IABP) [6]; hemodynamic parameters; biochemical markers; and echocardiographic measurements.

The hemodynamic parameters that can indicate RV failure after LVAD implantation include elevated preoperative and intraoperative central venous pressure (CVP) and reduced RV stroke work index (RVSWI<300 mmHg mL^{-1} m^{-2}) [4, 8, 21, 31]. Although high PAP is an easily measured parameter, RV function, which may not always be related to high PAP, remains the most critical determinant of survival. In fact, patients without pulmonary hypertension are more likely to develop RV failure and have more serious morbidity after LVAD implantation. This situation indicates that decreased RV contractility is unable to overcome increased PVR. RVAD or BiVAD support should be considered for patients with poor RV function indicated by low PAP or RVSWI. Preoperative treatment, including a pulmonary vasodilator, is required for patients with chronic pulmonary hypertension associated with pulmonary disease.

Findings consistent with organ failure and hepatic congestion secondary to impaired preoperative RV function are also important risk factors for postoperative RV failure and BiVAD requirement. These signs include elevated serum creatinine (Cr) [4, 31], blood urea nitrogen [8], aspartate aminotransferase (AST), and bilirubin levels [4]. Increased nonspecific neurohumoral markers of heart failure, such as N-terminal pro-brain natriuretic peptide and neopterin, and inflammatory markers such as procalcitonin and big endothelin-1 are also counted as risk factors for RV failure after LVAD implantation [24].

Severe preoperative TR and a short/long axis ratio of >0.6 for RV have high specificity (87 % and 97 %, respectively) and good sensitivity (66 % and 37 %) to identify patients with high risk of postoperative RV failure [9]. Increasing severity

Table 7.1 Risk score for mortality after LVAD implantation

Rao et al. [32]	
Preoperative variables	Weighting
Ventilated	4
Postcardiotomy	2
Pre-LVAD	2
CVP >16 mmHg	1
PT >16 s	1
Total points	Mortality (%)
Risk score	
>5	6
≤5	12

LVAD left ventricular assist device, *CVP* central venous pressure, *PT* prothrombin time

of TR is also associated with the occurrence of postoperative RV failure. Puwanant et al. found that preoperative TAPSE <7.5 mm was better related to post-LVAD RV failure than RVFAC, with a specificity of 91 % and a sensitivity of 46 % [28].

7.5.2 Risk Scores

Other risk scoring systems have been developed to quantify the risk of RV failure after LVAD implantation. Rao et al. revised a previous screening scale to more accurately predict survival after LVAD implantation and to determine emerging risk factors for mortality (Table 7.1). In their study, mechanical ventilation and a previous LVAD were independent predictors of mortality after device insertion. The correlation between observed and predicted values was better in the revised score than in the old score, which overpredicted mortality in patients at low risk and underpredicted mortality in patients at high risk [32].

Through multivariable regression analysis, Drakos et al. found seven preoperative variables that were correlated with postoperative RV failure, including destination therapy, IABP, and increased PVR [22] (Table 7.2). They reported that the incidence of postoperative RV failure was 44 %, although their study included various pulsatile and non-pulsatile LVAD systems. The authors defined RV failure as requirement for inotropic support for >14 days, *i*NO for >48 h, or RVAD implantation. Patients were stratified into four risk groups from a sum of all points assigned to each variable. The incidence of RV failure was 11 % in the lowest risk group, while in the highest group, it was 83 %. Destination therapy, elevated PVR, and preoperative IABP support were significant independent predictors for postoperative RV failure.

In a study with 197 patients undergoing LVAD, Matthews et al. reported that 35 % of the patients developed RV failure and that the independent predictors were the use of vasopressors and increased AST, bilirubin, and Cr levels; using these predictors, they developed a risk score system [4] (Table 7.2).

Table 7.2 Risk scores for RV failure after LVAD

Matthews et al. [4]		Drakos et al. [22]	
Preoperative variables	Points	Preoperative variables	Points
Vasopressor use	4	Destination therapy	3.5
Cr ≥2.3 mg/dL	3	IABP	4
Bilirubin ≥2 mg/dL	2.5	PVR	
AST ≥80 IU/L	2	1.7	1
		1.8–2.7	2
		2.8–4.2	3
		>4.3	4
		Inotrope dependency	2.5
		Obesity	2
		ACE or ARB	2.5
		β-blocker	2
Total points	Odds ratio	Total points	Risk (%)
Risk score for RV failure			
≤3.0	0.49	<5	11
4.0–5.0	2.8	5.5–8.0	37
≥5.5	7.6	8.5–12	56
		>12.5	83

RV right ventricle, *LVAD* left ventricular assist device, *Cr* creatinine, *AST* aspartate aminotransferase, *IABP* intra-aortic balloon pump, *PVR* pulmonary vascular resistance, *ACE* angiotensin-converting enzyme inhibitor, *ARB* angiotensin receptor blocker, *β-blocker* beta blocker

Fitzpatrick et al. proposed a similar risk score from a cohort of 266 patients after implantation of various types of LVAD [31]. In their study, they defined RV failure as the need for RVAD, which was found in 34 % of the patients. Using preoperative risk factors associated with postoperative RV failure, they proposed a risk score for RV failure based on multivariate logistic regression analysis. According to the scoring system, a score >50 is an indication for a BiVAD and has good sensitivity (83 %) and specificity (80 %).

The National Institutes of Health-sponsored Interagency Registry for Mechanical Assisted Circulatory Support (INTERMACS) developed a systematic scoring system through the largest LVAD database in the USA [33]. Alba et al. compared INTERMACS level I and II (sicker and decompensating) to level III and IV patients, showing that the system is a good predictor of postoperative complications and mortality, but not sensitive for postoperative RV failure [34].

7.6 Prevention and Management of RV Dysfunction

It is crucial to pay meticulous attention to optimizing preload, afterload, and contractility in patients with preexisting RV dysfunction in order to prevent RV failure (Fig. 7.2). Even simple measures such as maintenance of sinus rhythm or AV

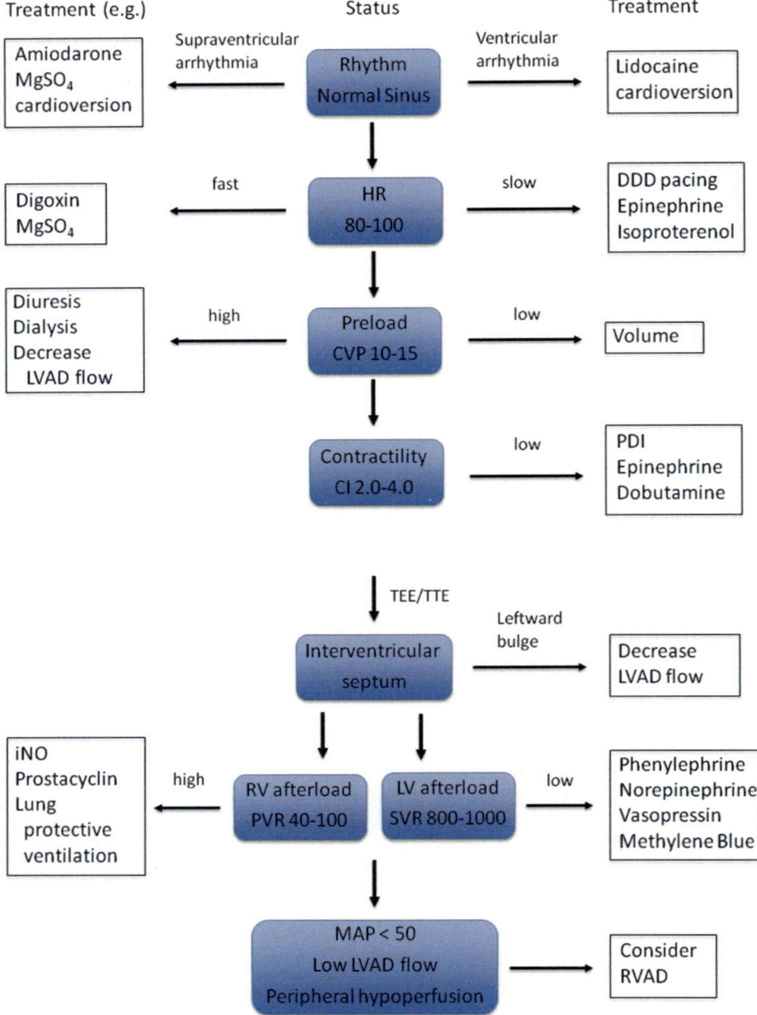

Fig. 7.2 Management algorithm for RVF. *RVF* right ventricular failure, *LVAD* left ventricular assist device, *MgSO₄* magnesium sulfate, *HR* heart rate (beat min⁻¹), *CVP* central venous pressure (mmHg), *CI* cardiac index (L min⁻¹ m⁻²), *PDI* phosphodiesterase inhibitor, *TEE* transesophageal echocardiography, TTE transthoracic echocardiography, *RV* right ventricle, *LV* left ventricle, *iNO* inhaled nitric oxide, *PVR* pulmonary vascular resistance (dyne s cm⁻⁵), *SVR* systemic vascular resistance (dyne s cm⁻⁵), *MAP* mean atrial pressure (mmHg), *RVAD* right ventricular assist device

synchronicity, adequate ventilation, temperature, and acid–base balance should be taken to prevent RV failure. Few studies have assessed the impact of preoperative management on post-LVAD RV failure.

7.6.1 Preoperative Prevention

Van Meter et al. developed an algorithm (Fig. 7.2) to prevent heart failure after LVAD implantation; this algorithm includes preoperative RV optimization and maintaining a CVP of <16 mmHg and a PA systolic pressure of <65 mmHg [30]. They proposed using RVAD support for patients with liver dysfunction, although their retrospective analysis of 35 pulsatile LVADs did not show the significance of this measure in preventing postoperative RV failure.

Although the optimal preoperative CVP is not well defined, some authors have found that CVP > 15 mmHg correlates to postoperative RV failure and requires further treatment [8, 30]. Aggressive preoperative diuresis, including hemodialysis if pharmacological treatment is not effective, is crucial to relieve RV distension, which is a grave predictor of perioperative RV failure [17].

Elevated PVR is one condition that mandates preoperative treatment for the management of perioperative heart failure [30]. Hemodynamic parameters obtained from the pulmonary artery catheter provide useful information for assessing PAP and PVR and for titrating pulmonary vasodilators.

Preoperative coagulopathy increases the risk of intraoperative bleeding that may necessitate blood transfusion, thus imposing an additional risk on RV function. Blood transfusion increases RV volume overload and PVR and may worsen SIRS; therefore, efforts are always made to minimize bleeding and the need for transfusion in every case. Preoperative use of vitamin K and intraoperative administration of aprotinin are common practices to reduce bleeding and thereby avoid excessive blood transfusion; these practices were confirmed efficient in studies of the first-generation LVAD systems [17, 35–37].

Pharmacological treatment of LV function is an important practice to maintain sufficient end-organ perfusion, thus minimizing hypotension and avoiding the vicious cycle of ischemia that further exacerbates heart failure. When pharmacological treatment is not effective, further measures that may include an IABP or even temporary mechanical support devices are considered [38]. Although preoperative IABP support is a risk factor for postoperative RV failure [6], on some occasions this practice may be an alternative because it could ultimately preserve RV function [39].

7.6.2 Pharmacological Management

Conventional therapy for LV dysfunction, such as introduction of a beta blockade or administration of angiotensin-converting enzyme inhibitors, is not always an ideal alternative for RV dysfunction. Instead, inotropes that induce a degree of pulmonary vasodilation, for example, dobutamine or milrinone, accompanied by inotropes that increase systolic blood pressure, i.e., epinephrine, for coronary perfusion, are more efficient for treatment for RV failure. Alpha-adrenergic stimulation may have a negative effect on RV function. Excessive contraction at the RV outflow tract (RVOT) may produce obstruction and decrease RV CO, especially when the RV is hypovolemic.

Specific pulmonary vasodilators, such as *i*NO and epoprostenol sodium, which reduce PVR and increase LVAD flow, are other important components of therapy in RV failure. Wagner et al. [40] studied the effect of up to 40 ppm *i*NO in patients with RV failure after LVAD implantation and reported that *i*NO significantly reduced PAP and PVR while increasing the cardiac index.

Vascular resistance can be reduced with the nitroso vasodilators such as nitro-glycerin, nitroprusside, and *i*NO, which increase levels of cyclic guanine mono-phosphate (cGMP) and cause smooth muscle relaxation and vasodilatation [41]. Although *i*NO is effective, its use is complicated by the inhaled delivery system and rebound pulmonary hypertension upon its withdrawal. Sildenafil is a type V phos-phodiesterase inhibitor that maintains cGMP levels and is effective for primary pul-monary hypertension [42]. Klodell et al. mentioned that sildenafil reduces PAP and averts rebound pulmonary hypertension [43].

Mortality is directly associated with the duration of inotropic support and remains high even after the inotropes are discontinued in patients with post-LVAD RV fail-ure. Schenk et al. reported that patients who tolerated early weaning from inotropes had better 6-month survival rates than those who did not [44].

7.6.3 Surgical Management

Preexisting native or prosthetic valve pathology does not affect the immediate post-operative mortality in patients with LVAD insertion. However, these valvular pathologies can complicate postoperative management in patients who are awaiting transplantation [45].

TR is considered a compensatory mechanism for an impaired RV and is not aggressively treated, even in patients with high risk of RV failure. However, after LVAD, functional TR may worsen because of the leftward-shifted IVS, with conse-quent tethering of the TV septal leaflet. Therefore, the degree of residual TR should be carefully evaluated intraoperatively by changing the LVAD flow after the patient is weaned from CPB. Correction of TR is an important procedure to decrease venous congestion, improve renal function, and further improve RV function. Criteria that have been proposed for TV repair during LVAD implantation include TV annulus >40 mm and moderate or severe TR [46–48].

Myocardial revascularization should also be considered to salvage hibernating RV myocardium [49]. Technical considerations, such as the relation of the LVAD outflow graft to right-sided structures may also influence RV function. We attempt to direct the outflow cannula lateral to the RA/RV to avoid compression when the chest is closed.

As a modification of the CPB technique, an RA to LA bypass or PA to aorta bypass may be an effective alternative to reduce RV overload and LV inflow [50, 51]. Off-pump LVAD implantation is also becoming popular, with advantages including reduced blood loss and avoidance of CPB-induced SIRS [52]. In addition, newly developed minimally invasive surgical techniques have advantages including diminished surgical stress and decreased postoperative morbidity [53].

Weaning from CPB is an important step to influence possible postoperative RV failure. Shortening CPB time, continuing ventilation during CPB, and minimizing blood transfusion and the attendant risk of lung injury are strategies that can avoid undesirable increases in PVR. Before weaning from CPB, careful de-airing of the heart under observation by transesophageal echocardiography (TEE) is essential to avoid systemic and right coronary air embolism. CO_2 insufflation in the surgical field has also been used to reduce air emboli [54]. In order to successfully wean a patient from CPB, CPB flow is gradually reduced in parallel with increase of LVAD flow under careful monitoring of RV function, LV volume, and IVS shift by TEE. An adequate LV volume is crucial to maintain the optimized IVS position. If the LV is underfilled, it will create a hazard because the IVS shifts towards the left side while LVAD flow increases to improve CO (suction cascade).

After discontinuation of CPB, a protective mechanical ventilation strategy with low PEEP, avoiding hypoxia and acidosis, should be used to maintain low PVR. The timing of protamine administration, which may cause an acute increase in PVR, should be carefully determined and should be deferred until hemodynamic stability is confirmed.

7.6.4 *Mechanical Support*

When RV failure occurs during surgery, weaning from CPB may be impossible, and alternative measures of mechanical support are taken. There is no report of long-term RVAD support, and RVAD support is recognized as a temporary rescue measure when conventional therapy for RV failure is unsuccessful. Although there are no established criteria for RVAD implantation, the largest study in the INTERMACS database reported that the incidence of postoperative RVAD implantation was 8 % in patients with LVAD, showing a poor outcome [55].

In a retrospective study, Fitzpatrick et al. reported that patients who underwent elective BiVAD implantation had better long-term survival than those who had emergent RVAD implant as support for acute RV failure after LVAD implantation [5]. Patients who needed BiVAD for severe RV failure had significantly poorer outcomes, characterized by high preoperative Cr and bilirubin levels, requirement for IABP support, lower RVSWI, and higher CVP and CVP/PCWP ratio.

Morgan et al. reported that patients who received early RVAD implantation during LVAD surgery had better survival than those with RVAD insertion >24 h after LVAD implantation [56]. On the other hand, patients who required RVAD after transplantation had reduced 1-, 5-, and 10-year survival rates compared to patients who did not require RVAD. In fact, RVAD implantation is an independent predictor of mortality in patients who receive an LVAD as BTT [8].

7.7 Conclusions

RV failure after LVAD implantation is a frequent and serious complication that increases mortality and morbidity. LVAD support has positive effects on the systemic circulation, but it may precipitate RV failure because of altered IVS position and increased RV preload, especially in patients with preexisting RV dysfunction. RV failure after LVAD implantation is multifactorial. Risk factors are found among patient characteristics, biochemical markers, and hemodynamic and echocardiographic parameters. These risk factors have been used to develop several risk scores for predicting potential post-LVAD RV failure.

To prevent RV failure after LVAD implantation, various measures should be taken. Preoperative management of RV function includes treatment of modifiable risk factors and optimization of RV preload and afterload while maintaining adequate end-organ perfusion. During surgery, minimizing blood transfusion and shortening CPB time are essential to avoid increasing PVR. In addition, surgical correction of TR may improve outcomes with decreased postoperative mortality and morbidity.

Although there is no established guideline for treatment of post-LVAD RV failure, postoperative mechanical support, including implantation of RVAD, is an alternative for RV failure refractory to medical treatment. There has also been some evidence that early introduction of RVAD or even elective BiVAD implantation during surgery improves outcomes.

References

1. Miller LW, Pagani FD, Russell SD, John R, Boyle AJ, Aaronson KD, et al. Use of a continuous-flow device in patients awaiting heart transplantation. N Engl J Med. 2007;357:885–96.
2. Slaughter MS, Rogers JG, Milano CA, Russell SD, Conte JV, Feldman D, et al. Advanced heart failure treated with continuous-flow left ventricular assist device. N Engl J Med. 2009;361:2241–51.
3. Pagani FD, Miller LW, Russell SD, Aaronson KD, John R, Boyle AJ, et al. Extended mechanical circulatory support with a continuous-flow rotary left ventricular assist device. J Am Coll Cardiol. 2009;54:312–21.
4. Matthews JC, Koelling TM, Pagani FD, Aaronson KD. The right ventricular failure risk score a preoperative tool for assessing the risk of right ventricular failure in left ventricular assist device candidates. J Am Coll Cardiol. 2008;51:2163–72.
5. Fitzpatrick 3rd JR, Frederick JR, Hsu VM, Hiesinger W, McCormick RC, Kozin ED, et al. Early planned institution of biventricular mechanical circulatory support results in improved outcomes compared with delayed conversion of a left ventricular assist device to a biventricular assist device. J Thorac Cardiovasc Surg. 2009;137:971–7.
6. Patel ND, Weiss ES, Schaffer J, Ullrich SL, Rivard DC, Shah AS et al. Right heart dysfunction after left ventricular assist device implantation: a comparison of the pulsatile Heart Mate I and axial-flow Heart Mate II devices. Ann Thorac Surg. 2008;86:832–40. Discussion – 40.
7. Hennig F, Stepanenko AV, Lehmkuhl HB, Kukucka M, Dandel M, Krabatsch T, et al. Neurohumoral and inflammatory markers for prediction of right ventricular failure after implantation of a left ventricular assist device. Gen Thorac Cardiovasc Surg. 2009;59:19–24.

8. Kormos RL, Teuteberg JJ, Pagani FD, Russell SD, John R, Miller LW, et al. Right ventricular failure in patients with the HeartMate II continuous-flow left ventricular assist device: incidence, risk factors, and effect on outcomes. J Thorac Cardiovasc Surg. 2010;139:1316–24.

9. Baumwol J, Macdonald PS, Keogh AM, Kotlyar E, Spratt P, Jansz P, et al. Right heart failure and "failure to thrive" after left ventricular assist device: clinical predictors and outcomes. J Heart Lung Transplant. 2011;30:888–95.

10. Santambrogio L, Bianchi T, Fuardo M, Gazzoli F, Veronesi R, Braschi A, et al. Right ventricular failure after left ventricular assist device insertion: preoperative risk factors. Interact Cardiovasc Thorac Surg. 2006;5:379–82.

11. Haddad F, Hunt SA, Rosenthal DN, Murphy DJ. Right ventricular function in cardiovascular disease, part I: anatomy, physiology, aging, and functional assessment of the right ventricle. Circulation. 2008;117:1436–48.

12. Voelkel NF, Quaife RA, Leinwand LA, Barst RJ, McGoon MD, Meldrum DR, et al. Right ventricular function and failure: report of a National Heart, Lung, and Blood Institute working group on cellular and molecular mechanisms of right heart failure. Circulation. 2006;114:1883–91.

13. Lorenz CH, Walker ES, Morgan VL, Klein SS, Graham Jr TP. Normal human right and left ventricular mass, systolic function, and gender differences by cine magnetic resonance imaging. J Cardiovasc Magn Reson. 1999;1:7–21.

14. Walker LA, Buttrick PM. The right ventricle: biologic insights and response to disease. Curr Cardiol Rev. 2009;5:22–8.

15. Kevin LG, Barnard M. Right ventricular failure. Oxford J. 2007;7(3):89–94.

16. Pfisterer M. Right ventricular involvement in myocardial infarction and cardiogenic shock. Lancet. 2003;362:392–4.

17. John R, Lee S, Eckman P, Liao K. Right ventricular failure–a continuing problem in patients with left ventricular assist device support. J Cardiovasc Transl Res. 2010;3:604–11.

18. Thunberg CA, Gaitan BD, Arabia FA, Cole DJ, Grigore AM. Ventricular assist devices today and tomorrow. J Cardiothorac Vasc Anesth. 2010;24:656–80.

19. Lee S, Kamdar F, Madlon-Kay R, Boyle A, Colvin-Adams M, Pritzker M, et al. Effects of the Heart Mate II continuous-flow left ventricular assist device on right ventricular function. J Heart Lung Transplant. 2010;29:209–15.

20. Greyson CR. Pathophysiology of right ventricular failure. Crit Care Med. 2008 Jan;36(1 Suppl):S57–65.

21. Dang NC, Topkara VK, Mercando M, Kay J, Kruger KH, Aboodi MS, et al. Right heart failure after left ventricular assist device implantation in patients with chronic congestive heart failure. J Heart Lung Transplant. 2006;25:1–6.

22. Drakos SG, Janicki L, Horne BD, Kfoury AG, Reid BB, Clayson S, et al. Risk factors predictive of right ventricular failure after left ventricular assist device implantation. Am J Cardiol. 2010;105:1030–5.

23. Ochiai Y, McCarthy PM, Smedira NG, Banbury MK, Navia JL, Feng J, et al. Predictors of severe right ventricular failure after implantable left ventricular assist device insertion: analysis of 245 patients. Circulation. 2002;106(12 Suppl. 1):I198–I202.

24. Potapov EV, Stepanenko A, Dandel M, Kukucka M, Lehmkuhl HB, Weng Y, et al. Tricuspid incompetence and geometry of the right ventricle as predictors of right ventricular function after implantation of a left ventricular assist device. J Heart Lung Transplant. 2008;27:1275–81.

25. Rudski LG, Lai WW, Afilalo J, Hua L, Handschumacher MD, Chandrasekaran K, et al. Guidelines for the echocardiographic assessment of the right heart in adults: a report from the American Society of Echocardiography endorsed by the European Association of Echocardiography, a registered branch of the European Society of Cardiology, and the Canadian Society of Echocardiography. J Am Soc Echocardiogr. 2010;23:685–713. quiz 86–8.

26. Mertens LL, Friedberg MK. Imaging the right ventricle–current state of the art. Nat Rev Cardiol. 2010;7:551–63.

27. Estep JD, Stainback RF, Little SH, Torre G, Zoghbi WA. The role of echocardiography and other imaging modalities in patients with left ventricular assist devices. JACC Cardiovasc Imaging. 2010;3:1049–64.

28. Puwanant S, Hamilton KK, Klodell CT, Hill JA, Schofield RS, Cleeton TS, et al. Tricuspid annular motion as a predictor of severe right ventricular failure after left ventricular assist device implantation. J Heart Lung Transplant. 2008;27:1102–7.

29. Meineri M, Van Rensburg AE, Vegas A. Right ventricular failure after LVAD implantation: prevention and treatment. Best Pract Res Clin Anaesthesiol. 2012;26:217–29.

30. Van Meter Jr CH. Right heart failure: best treated by avoidance. Ann Thorac Surg. 2001;71 (3 Suppl):S220–2.

31. Fitzpatrick 3rd JR, Frederick JR, Hsu VM, Kozin ED, O'Hara ML, Howell E, et al. Risk score derived from pre-operative data analysis predicts the need for biventricular mechanical circulatory support. J Heart Lung Transplant. 2008;27:1286–92.

32. Rao V, Oz MC, Flannery MA, Catanese KA, Argenziano M, Naka Y. Revised screening scale to predict survival after insertion of a left ventricular assist device. J Thorac Cardiovasc Surg. 2003;125:855–62.

33. Kirklin JK, Naftel DC, Stevenson LW, Kormos RL, Pagani FD, Miller MA, et al. INTERMACS database for durable devices for circulatory support: first annual report. J Heart Lung Transplant. 2008;27:1065–72.

34. Alba AC, Rao V, Ivanov J, Ross HJ, Delgado DH. Usefulness of the INTERMACS scale to predict outcomes after mechanical assist device implantation. J Heart Lung Transplant. 2009;28:827–33.

35. Kaplon RJ, Gillinov AM, Smedira NG, Kottke-Marchant K, Wang IW, Goormastic M, et al. Vitamin K reduces bleeding in left ventricular assist device recipients. J Heart Lung Transplant. 1999;18:346–50.

36. Goldstein DJ, Seldomridge JA, Chen JM, Catanese KA, DeRosa CM, Weinberg AD, et al. Use of aprotinin in LVAD recipients reduces blood loss, blood use, and perioperative mortality. Ann Thorac Surg. 1995 May;59:1063–67. Discussion 8.

37. Morgan JA, John R, Rao V, Weinberg AD, Lee BJ, Mazzeo PA, et al. Bridging to transplant with the HeartMate left ventricular assist device: the Columbia Presbyterian 12-year experience. J Thorac Cardiovasc Surg. 2004;127:1309–16.

38. Neuzil P, Kmonicek P, Skoda J, Reddy VY. Temporary [short-term] percutaneous left ventricular assist device [Tandem Heart] in a patient with STEMI, multivessel coronary artery disease, cardiogenic shock and severe peripheral artery disease. Acute Card Care. 2009;11:146–50.

39. Boeken U, Feindt P, Litmathe J, Kurt M, Gams E. Intraaortic balloon pumping in patients with right ventricular insufficiency after cardiac surgery: parameters to predict failure of IABP Support. J Thorac Cardiovasc Surg. 2009;57:324–8.

40. Wagner F, Dandel M, Gunther G, Loebe M, Schulze-Neick I, Laucke U et al. Nitric oxide inhalation in the treatment of right ventricular dysfunction following left ventricular assist device implantation. Circulation 1997; 96: II–6.

41. Haddad E, Lowson SM, Johns RA, Rich GF. Use of inhaled nitric oxide perioperatively and in intensive care patients. Anesthesiology. 2000;92:1821–5.

42. Prasad S, Wilkinson J, Gatzoulis MA. Sildenafil in primary pulmonary hypertension. N Engl J Med. 2000;343:1342.

43. Klodell Jr CT, Morey TE, Lobato EB, Aranda Jr JM, Staples ED, Schofield RS, et al. Effect of sildenafil on pulmonary artery pressure, systemic pressure, and nitric oxide utilization in patients with left ventricular assist devices. Ann Thorac Surg. 2007;83:68–71.

44. SchenkS, McCarthy PM, Blackstone EH, et al. Duration of inotropic support after left ventricular assist device implantation: risk factors and impact on outcome. J Thorac Cardiovasc Surg 2006; 131: 447–54.

45. Rao V, Slater JP, Edwards NM, Naka Y, Oz MC. Surgical management of valvular disease in patients requiring left ventricular assist device support. Ann Thorac Surg. 2001;71:1448–53.

46. Krishan K, Nair A, Pinney S, Adams DH, Anyanwu AC. Liberal use of tricuspid-valve annuloplasty during left-ventricular assist device implantation. Eur J Cardiothorac Surg. 2012;41:213–7.

47. Piacentino 3rd V, Troupes CD, Ganapathi AM, Blue LJ, Mackensen GB, Swaminathan M, et al. Clinical impact of concomitant tricuspid valve procedures during left ventricular assist device implantation. Ann Thorac Surg. 2011;92:1414–8. Discussion 8–9.

48. Maltais S, Topilsky Y, Tchantchaleishvili V, McKellar SH, Durham LA, Joyce LD, et al. Surgical treatment of tricuspid valve insufficiency promotes early reverse remodeling in patients with axial-flow left ventricular assist devices. J Thorac Cardiovasc Surg. 2012;143: 1370–76.
49. Potapov EV, Sodian R, Loebe M, Drews T, Dreysse S, Hetzer R. Revascularization of the occluded right coronary artery during left ventricular assist device implantation. J Heart Lung Transplant. 2001;20:918–22.
50. Van Meter Jr CH, Robbins RJ, Ochsner JL. Technique of right heart protection and deairing during HeartMate vented electric LVAD implantation. Ann Thorac Surg. 1997;63:1191–2.
51. Loebe M, Potapov E, Sodian R, Kopitz M, Noon GP. A safe and simple method of preserving right ventricular function during implantation of a left ventricular assist device. J Thorac Cardiovasc Surg. 2001;122:1043.
52. Sun BC, Firstenberg MS, Louis LB, Panza A, Crestanello JA, Sirak J, et al. Placement of long-term implantable ventricular assist devices without the use of cardiopulmonary bypass. J Heart Lung Transplant. 2008;27:718–21.
53. Ghodsizad A, Kar BJ, Layolka P, Okur A, Gonzales J, Bara C, et al. Less invasive off-pump implantation of axial flow pumps in chronic ischemic heart failure: survival effects. J Heart Lung Transplant. 2011;30:834–7.
54. Woo YJ, Acker MA. Implantable ventricular assist device exchange with focused intravascular deairing techniques. Ann Thorac Surg. 2011;91:306–7.
55. Kirklin JK, Naftel DC, Kormos RL, Stevenson LW, Pagani FD, Miller MA, et al. Third INTERMACS annual report: the evolution of destination therapy in the United States. J Heart Lung Transplant. 2011;30:115–23.
56. Morgan JA, John R, Lee BJ, Oz MC, Naka Y. Is severe right ventricular failure in left ventricular assist device recipients a risk factor for unsuccessful bridging to transplant and post-transplant mortality. Ann Thorac Surg. 2004;77:859–63.

Chapter 8
Innovation Update

David J. Farrar, Kevin Bourque, Steven H. Reichenbach,
Paul Muller, and Laxmi Peri

Abstract There have been significant advancements in continuous-flow left ventricular assist devices over the past few years, but new devices are still needed to improve the quality of life of patients with advanced heart failure and reduce adverse events. In this chapter we describe a fully magnetically levitated left ventricular assist device (HeartMate III), a fully implanted left ventricular assist system with the percutaneous driveline replaced by a wireless energy transmission system for tether-free support (FILVAS), an ultraminiaturized VAD (the HeartMate X) for left, right, or biventricular support, and a new percutaneous heart pump (HeartMate PHP) to address needs for patients needing short-term hemodynamic support.

Keywords Magnetically levitated LVAD • Transcutaneous power transmission • Expandable percutaneous catheter pump

8.1 Introduction

Over the last decade there have been significant improvements in clinical outcomes in patients implanted with continuous-flow left ventricular assist devices compared to the first-generation pulsatile-flow devices. With this increasing experience, one-year survival rates with the HeartMate II LVAS have increased to 85 % for bridge to transplantation [1–3] and to 73 % for destination therapy [4], compared to only 55 % survival for patients receiving the HeartMate XVE pulsatile-flow left ventricular assist device (LVAD) [5]. In addition, adverse event rates for the continuous-flow

D.J. Farrar (✉) • K. Bourque • S.H. Reichenbach • P. Muller • L. Peri
Thoratec Corporation, 6035 Stoneridge Dr Pleasanton,
California, CA 94556, USA
e-mail: david.farrar@thoratec.com

S. Kyo (ed.), *Ventricular Assist Devices in Advanced-Stage Heart Failure*,
DOI 10.1007/978-4-431-54466-1_8, © Springer Japan 2014

HeartMate II LVADs were better than the pulsatile-flow LVAD for most categories [5], and hemorrhagic stroke and driveline infection rates have further declined [4]. Over 15,000 patients have been implanted with the HeartMate II LVAS and patients have been supported for over 8 years.

However, in spite of these clinical and technological advances, there is still a need to improve quality of life of patients with long-term mechanical circulatory support devices and to further reduce adverse events. In this chapter we discuss the status of several new mechanical circulatory support devices to meet these needs.[1]

8.2 HeartMate III

The HeartMate III LVAD is a compact centrifugal pump with a fully magnetically levitated rotor targeting optimal hemocompatibility (Fig. 8.1). This LVAD, substantially miniaturized since previous descriptions of an earlier prototype [6, 7], is part of a long-term, full support (up to 10 L/min) system designed to enhance surgery, reduce MCS adverse events, and improve patient quality of life.

The rotor is fully supported by magnetic levitation, obviating mechanical or fluid bearings. Both drive (i.e., rotation) and levitation of the rotor are accomplished using a single stator comprising iron poles, copper coils, and position sensors. By measuring the position of a permanent magnet in the rotor and appropriately controlling the current in the drive and levitation coils, the radial position and rotational

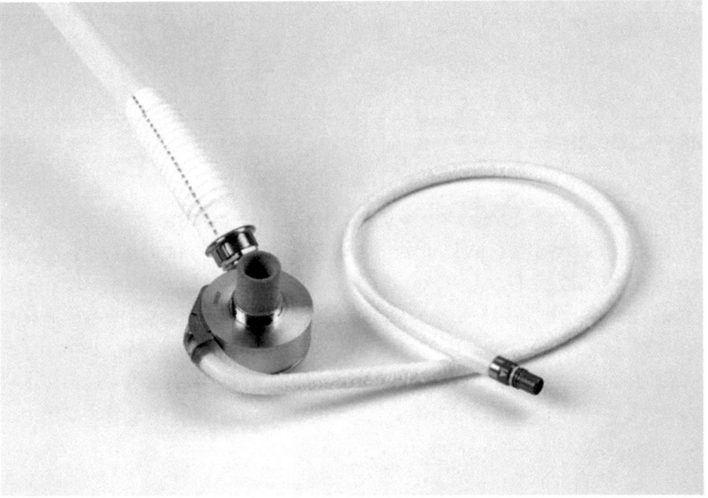

Fig. 8.1 HeartMate III fully magnetically levitated left ventricular assist system

---

[1] All devices in this chapter are in development and not in clinical use as of June 2013.

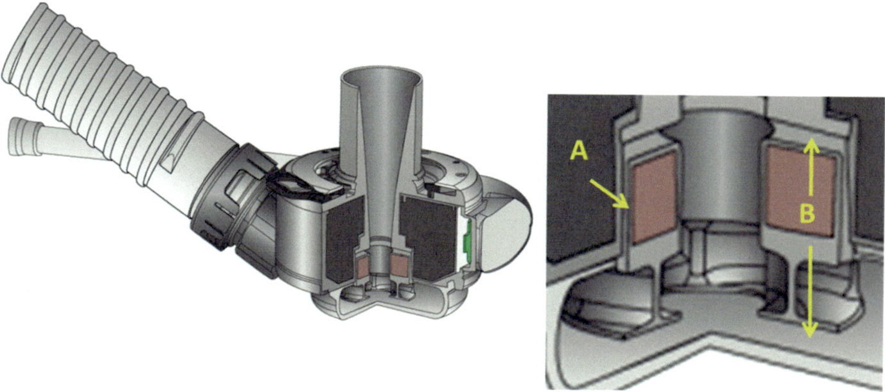

Fig. 8.2 Cross section of HeartMate III LVAD. Wide gaps for secondary flow paths of 0.5 mm radially (**a**) to 1.0 mm axially (**b**) are possible with full magnetic levitation design

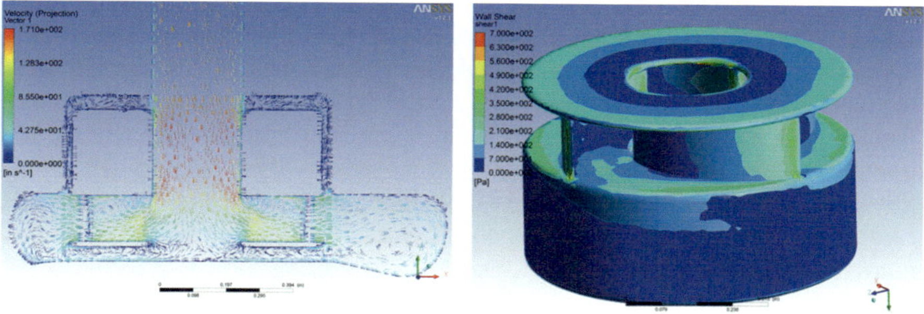

Fig. 8.3 Computational fluid dynamics (CFD) analysis of HeartMate III blood pump illustrates low shear, well-organized flow fields, smooth flow transitions, and the avoidance of regions of stasis over wide ranges of flow

speed of the rotor are actively and independently controlled. Because of the permanent magnet's attraction to the iron pole pieces, the rotor passively resists excursion in the axial direction, whether translating or tilting.

This magnetic levitation technology essentially eliminates rotor mechanical wear as a reliability factor and facilitates relatively large gaps between the turning rotor and the stationary housing (Fig. 8.2). These gaps are approximately 0.5 mm radially and 1.0 mm axially, 10–20 times greater than those in a hydrodynamic bearing. Computational fluid dynamic (CFD) analysis confirms that flow fields are well organized across wide ranges of flow (2–10 L/min) and that surface shear forces are kept lower than other types of pumps (Fig. 8.3). An additional benefit of magnetic levitation is that these large gaps are maintained irrespective of rotor speed, even when not turning. Thus, it is conceivable to operate at lower speeds, which might be important in future applications such as partial left ventricular assistance, right ventricular assistance, or weaning exercises.

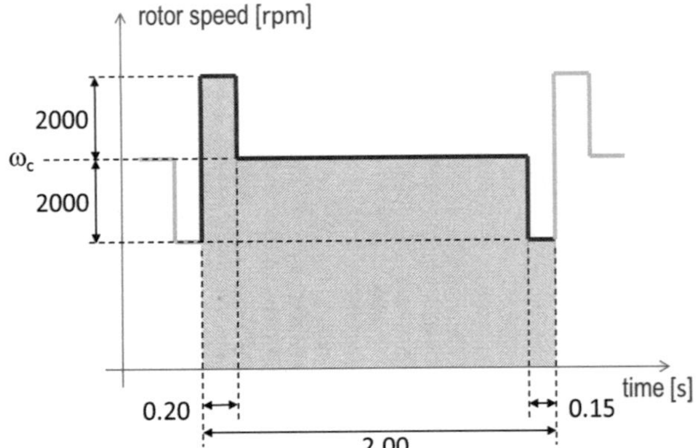

Fig. 8.4 Schematic of the changes in rotor speed above and below the set speed w_c to create the HeartMate III artificial pulse

In blood, large gaps are advantageous in several ways. Low hydraulic resistance ensures avoidance of stasis in those regions. Low shear stresses reduce trauma to erythrocytes and circulating proteins, which could beneficially affect adverse events such as thromboembolism, hemolysis, and bleeding. Further, because minor radial and axial deviation of the rotor is tolerable, levitation is readily maintained through the most rigorous patient activities, and a novel feature called an artificial pulse is facilitated. As for other rotary pumps, with HeartMate III the clinician will set only a single speed, w_c in Fig. 8.4; however, the rotor speed will periodically depart from this value in order to contribute a flow disruption that in some ways mimics native cardiac contractility. This artificial pulse "beats" 30 times per minute, asynchronously with the heart.

Although it has been well established with continuous-flow LVADs that an MCS device does not need to pulse for survival, there are theoretical advantages in contributing or enhancing the native pulsatility in various conditions [6]. Indeed, there are distinct benefits in producing unsteadiness in the flow within any rotary pump, and there may be similar benefits external to the pump, reducing adverse events such as aortic insufficiency and bleeding, for example.

To further optimize hemocompatibility, in addition to reducing shear and increasing washing, all the blood-contacting titanium surfaces except for the rotor and rotor well are coated with sintered titanium microspheres. Surfaces textured in this fashion in HeartMates XVE and II have been shown to promote the growth of a stable, adherent biological lining that reduces thromboembolic risk and the level of required anticoagulation therapy.

The electronics and software necessary to control motor drive and levitation are integrated into the implantable motor, and miniaturization was a major focus to make the LVAD as small as possible. Several important design features, including a low-profile apical sewing cuff and quick-connect attachment mechanism, minimize the effective size of the LVAD, and validation studies have shown that the LVAD is readily implanted in the thorax, obviating a pump pocket.

The magnetic levitation technology to achieve the hemocompatibility benefits includes implanted electronics which minimize the number of electrical conductors in the percutaneous cable and stage the LVAD for a future fully implanted configuration, i.e., with no percutaneous lead (see next section). For now, the HeartMate III percutaneous cable has been constructed with an armor layer for damage resistance and features an inline connector that permits a smaller tunneling core and replacement of the external portion without pump replacement if necessary.

The combination of features addressing hemocompatibility (large pump gaps, low shear stress, artificial pulse, and textured blood-contacting surfaces), surgical implantation (small size, engineered apical attachment, and modular driveline), and reduced power consumption is expected to result in an advance in MCS outcomes: lower adverse events and higher patient quality of life.

8.3 Fully Implanted Left Ventricular Assist System

Although there have been HeartMate II patients successfully supported for more than 8 years with a percutaneous lead, it is clear that for maximum freedom from infection and for improved physical and psychological quality of life, a system without percutaneous leads is highly desirable. To meet this need, a fully implanted LVAD system (FILVAS) with transcutaneous energy transmission is in development. We envision a system that would allow a flexible lifestyle with mobile, tethered, and free operation modes (Fig. 8.5) by eliminating the driveline and "around the clock"

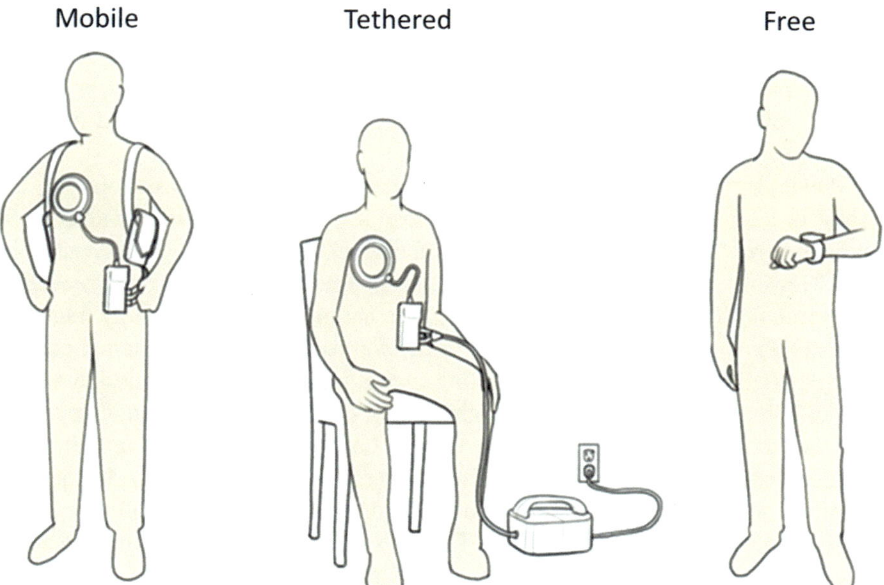

Fig. 8.5 Different configurations for use of the HeartMate fully implanted system (FILVAS). Mobile: Patient in mobile configuration with wearable external batteries and power transmission components for typical mobile use. Tethered: Patient tethered to external power module connected to line power, typically for sleeping and stationary use. Free: Patient in untethered mode with LVAD powered by internal batteries, free from any external equipment. Monitoring of internal device function is achieved with wrist monitor

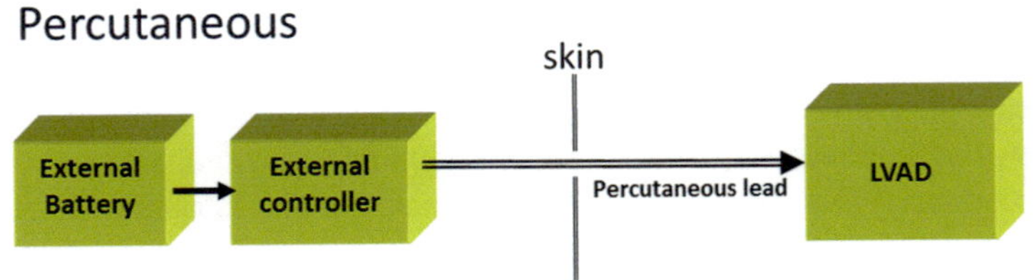

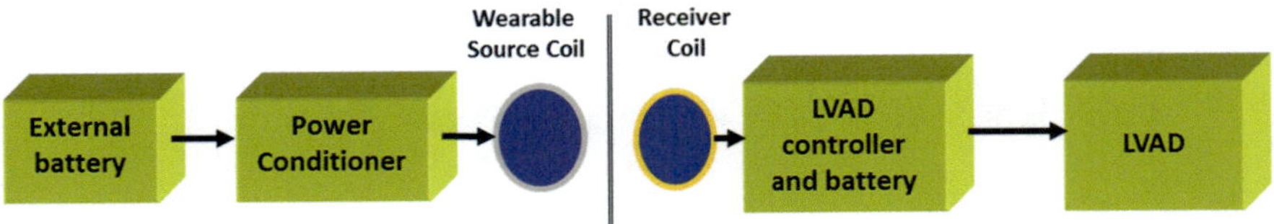

Fig. 8.6 Comparison of LVAD system with percutaneous lead and with transcutaneous energy transmission. Resonant energy transmission system enables high-efficiency, user-friendly wireless energy transfer across wider distances than with previous designs. Magnetic fields of the two coils couple tightly. AC power through the source coil induces a magnetic field, which induces current in the implanted power capture coil

worn equipment necessary with a percutaneous lead system. Components necessary to eliminate the percutaneous lead include external power conditioner, wearable source coil and internal receiver coil, implanted LVAD controller, and batteries (Fig. 8.6).

Previous clinical experience with transcutaneous energy transmission with the AbioCor total artificial heart and the LionHeart left ventricular assist systems [8, 9] provided proof of principle and illustrated the benefits of not having a percutaneous lead. However, these early systems also illustrated several limitations that needed to be overcome. These systems required the external transcutaneous energy transmission (TET) coil to be well aligned and in close proximity with the internal coil for energy transfer. With this close coupling requirement, power transmission was at risk of being disrupted by positional changes or even weight gain. Another limitation was the implanted battery which allowed only a limited amount of tether-free run time, as little as 30 min, and it needed to be replaced too frequently. Major technological advances over the last few years provide the opportunity for fully implanted systems to realize their full potential. These advances include new wireless energy transfer technology and improvements in implanted battery technology.

Incorporating a new nonradiative resonant magnetic coupling approach into a TETS has allowed high-efficiency, alignment tolerant wireless energy transfer capable of power transfer across much wider distances than was achieved with previous designs. This approach utilizes near-field strong coupling modes that arise between

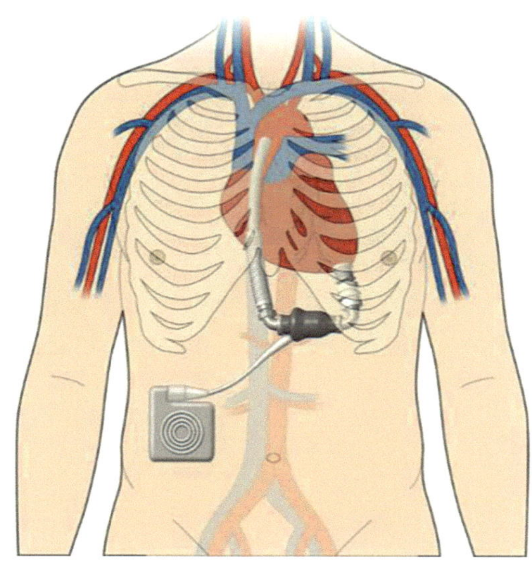

Fig. 8.7 Illustration showing the implanted components of the fully implanted left ventricular assist system (FILVAS). The LVAD is powered by an implanted unit which includes the power receiver coil, implanted batteries, and pump controller

two high-efficiency resonators tuned to close but unequal frequencies and separated by distances comparable to their size [11]. It also makes use of high magnetic permeability materials in the resonator construction to concentrate the transmitted magnetic flux where it can be captured by the implanted receiver, significantly reducing the deleterious effects of coil misalignment experienced in earlier designs.

Robust battery technology tailored for implantable LVAD application, which is expected to provide substantially longer tether-free operation for the patient and to extend the expected battery replacement interval beyond 3 years due to the high charge–discharge cycle life of the new battery chemistry.

The fully implanted components (Fig. 8.7) are in development to provide platform technologies that can be designed to work with any LVAD, especially the HeartMate II, HeartMate III, or HeartMate X. It is envisioned that the first fully implanted system will be with the HeartMate II because of the extensive clinical experience and proven track record as an LVAD in percutaneous applications.

8.4 HeartMate X

There are other clinical needs that will be addressed with the HeartMate X. This ultracompact, highly versatile VAD is designed to address the needs of two distinct patient populations including much earlier stage heart failure patients and those with biventricular failure. This blood pump (Fig. 8.8) is designed to provide partial to full circulatory support in an ultracompact size, typically expected to be used in the 3–5 L/min range. The design envelope used for maximizing efficiency and

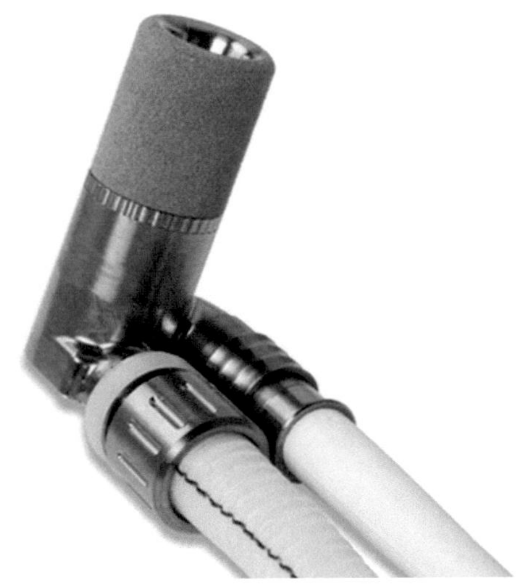

Fig. 8.8 The HeartMate X is a miniaturized blood pump utilizing proven bearing technology from the HeartMate II LVAD and is designed for LVAD, RVAD, and BiVAD use. The very compact package is about the same total size as the inflow conduit in the HeartMate II

hemocompatibility is extended between 2.5 L/min for partial support, 5.3 L/min for nominal full support (the average flow of current HeartMate II patients), and 4.3 L/min for right-sided support, but with capability to achieve 8 L/min. The HeartMate X utilizes the HeartMate II blood-immersed bearing technology which has proven to be extremely robust and durable in clinical use with the estimated bearing life greatly exceeding 17 years [10].

In addition to the hemocompatible and durable design, expanding the application to substantially less-sick heart failure patients needing only partial support requires peripherals that are smaller, lighter, and easier to use for improved patient quality of life. The HeartMate X has been designed to be highly power efficient, so the size and weight of the external electronic components can be minimized and battery run times can be maximized. A substantially smaller controller incorporating an internal battery was designed for the system (140 g; 160 mm^3) (Fig. 8.9). In its minimal-use configuration this small single component of the controller provides over 2 h of run time under partial support conditions. With an attachable extended-use battery pack the system provides over 8 h of run time under the same conditions.

The expected benefits of this technology include options for minimally invasive implantation as well as the versatility for use in LVAD, in RVAD, or for BiVAD support. With a pump body diameter of 2.2 cm, the pump is designed to facilitate non-sternotomy implant approaches via thoracotomy or subcostal incisions. Similarly, the outflow was designed to accommodate multiple configurations and pump positions including options for implantation without cardiopulmonary bypass. The small pump size also allows for versatility in biventricular cannulation approaches (Fig. 8.10) including the LVAD connected from LV to the aorta and the RVAD with either right atrial or right ventricular cannulation on the diaphragmatic surface of the RV free wall, with blood flow return to the pulmonary artery.

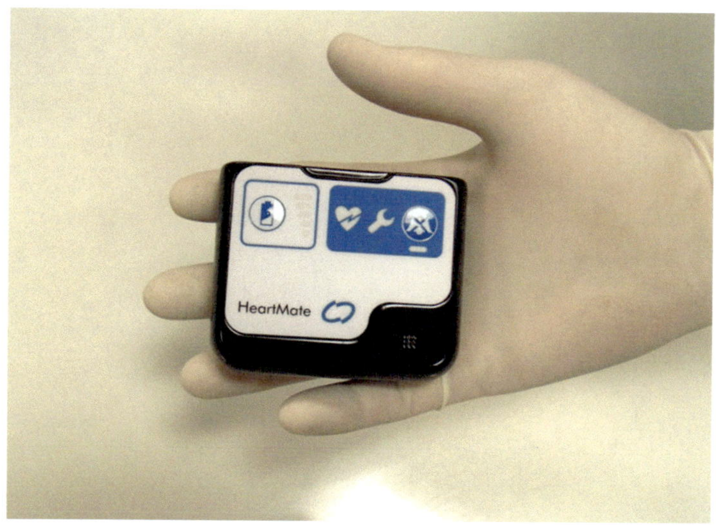

Fig. 8.9 Miniature standalone HeartMate X controller with internal battery

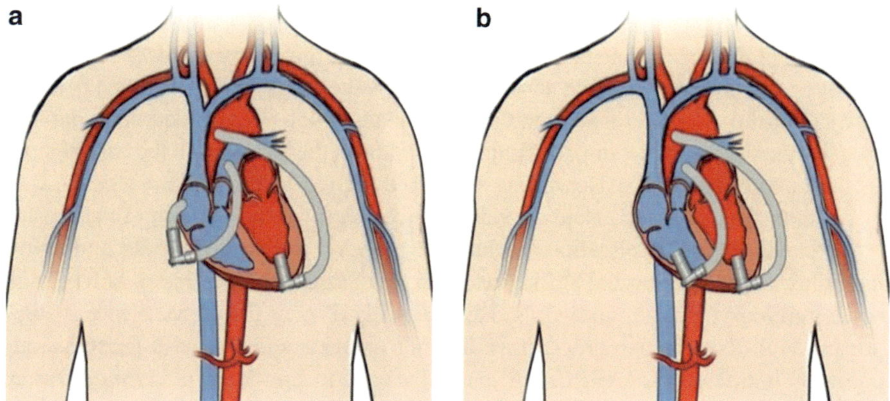

Fig. 8.10 Options for biventricular placement of HeartMate X miniaturized blood pumps. (**a**) LVAD with LV to aorta cannulation and RVAD with right atrial to pulmonary artery cannulation; (**b**) same but with right ventricular cannulation for the RVAD on the diaphragmatic surface of the RV free wall

8.5   HeartMate Percutaneous Heart Pump

The HeartMate percutaneous heart pump (PHP) system (Fig. 8.11) is a catheter-based heart pump and console designed to provide hemodynamic left ventricular support for up to multiple days to maintain adequate systemic cardiac output. The key feature of the HeartMate PHP is its ability to be deployed percutaneously via an integrated

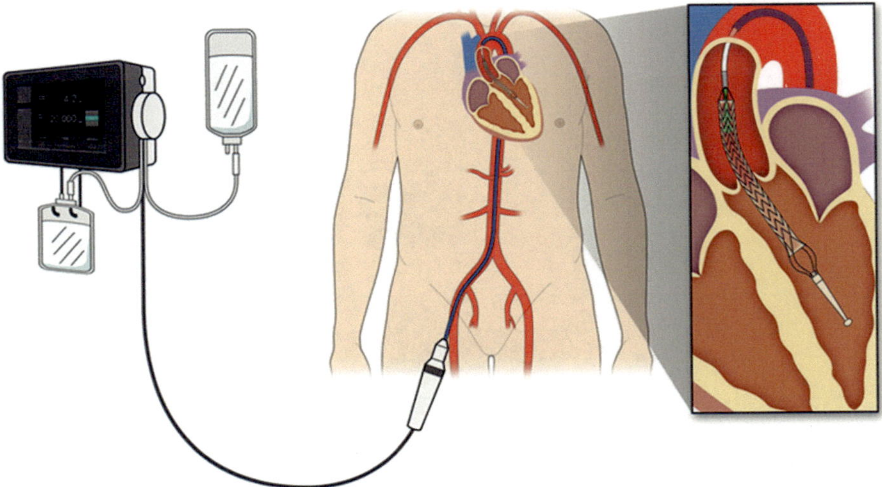

Fig. 8.11 Illustration showing HeartMate PHP operational mode. Introduced via the femoral artery across the aortic valve with sheath fully withdrawn allowing expansion of the elastomeric impeller and nitinol cannula

13 F arterial sheath. The distal portion of the catheter then expands to 24 F after it is deployed into the left ventricle across the aortic valve. This feature is made possible by a collapsible impeller and cannula mechanism, which is expanded upon deployment by the operator. The impeller pumps blood from the LV through the cannula into the ascending aorta. The HeartMate PHP is designed to provide average flow of 4–5 L/min. An external console provides device control and monitoring functions.

Potential clinical applications include cardiogenic shock of multiple etiologies, including acute myocardial infarction, decompensated chronic heart failure, and acute cardiomyopathy/myocarditis. HeartMate PHP may also have a role in supporting high-risk elective procedures, like VT ablation and high-risk percutaneous coronary interventions (HRPCI). It is ideally used to provide rapid hemodynamic stabilization of patients with compromised acute or acute-on-chronic ventricular deterioration. This will provide sufficient time for either patient recovery or to make clinical decisions regarding advanced surgical management, including options for bridging to long-term LVAD support. Figure 8.12 (middle) shows the PHP in the sheath and partially and fully unsheathed. The sheathed PHP is inserted via the femoral artery and threaded across the aortic valve (left), and removal of the sheath allows expansion of the device for operation (right). At the end of the support period, the cannula is re-sheathed, and the catheter pump is removed through the initial insertion site.

The first-in-human experience with HeartMate PHP occurred in March 2013 at Sanatorio Italiano in Paraguay. Three patients with multivessel coronary disease

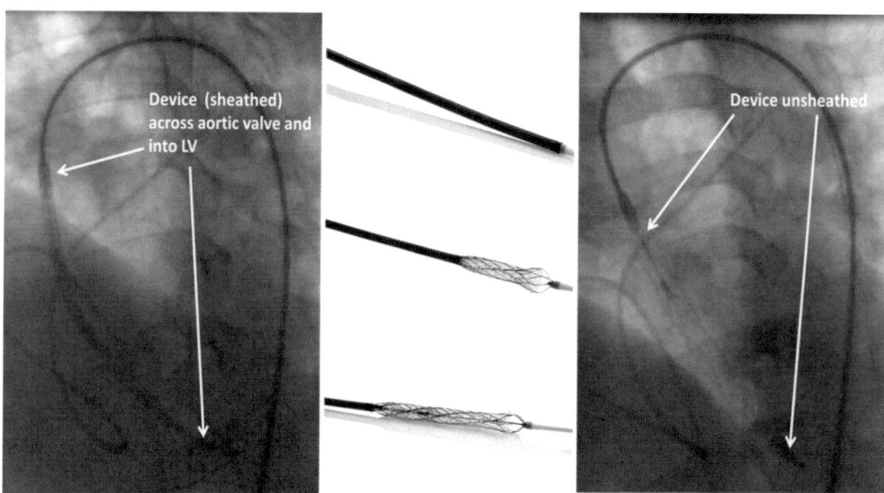

Fig. 8.12 HeartMate PHP sheathed for insertion across the aortic valve and into the left ventricle (*left*). PHP in the sheath, and partially and fully unsheathed (*middle*), PHP with the outer sheath withdrawn showing the collapsible elastomeric impeller and nitinol cannula in the expanded operational state (*right*)

and reduced LV function underwent elective PCI. Ejection fraction ranged from 26 to 34 %. Major adverse events (death, MI, CVA/TIA, limb ischemia, vascular complications, aortic valve insufficiency) were evaluated during PHP use, in-hospital and at 30-day follow-up. Intraprocedural evaluations included device success, defined as the successful deployment, use and removal of PHP without device failure, and the measurement of hemodynamics at baseline and during support. Baseline, periprocedural, and 30-day echocardiography were performed to assess for aortic valve abnormalities or regurgitation. Ejection fraction was verified at baseline using echocardiography. Device placement occurred through the left femoral artery via a standard introducer. Right heart catheterization was performed to obtain hemodynamic measurements.

The device was successfully deployed in all patients without complications. There was no periprocedural or follow-up echocardiographic evidence of aortic regurgitation or valve abnormalities. All planned target lesions were revascularized. The device was successfully removed in all cases. Hemodynamic measurements were obtained prior to device use and during device support.

The feasibility of using the HeartMate PHP was demonstrated in a small first-in-human cohort. This novel device was safely and successfully used without adverse patient events. All patients were discharged between 24 and 48 h of PCI and were clinically stable through the 30-day follow-up period. Further studies and formal clinical trials are planned to evaluate the HeartMate PHP in high-risk PCI and other patient populations.

References

1. Starling RC, Naka Y, Boyle AJ, Gonzalez-Stawinski G, John R, Jorde U, Russell SD, Conte JV, Aaronson KD, McGee Jr EC, Cotts WG, DeNofrio D, Pham DT, Farrar DJ, Pagani FD. Results of the post-U.S. Food and Drug Administration-approval study with a continuous flow left ventricular assist device as a bridge to heart transplantation: a prospective study using INTERMACS. J Am Coll Cardiol. 2011;57(19):1890–8.
2. John R, Naka Y, Smedira NG, Starling R, Jorde U, Eckman P, Farrar DJ, Pagani FD. Continuous flow left ventricular assist device outcomes in commercial use compared with the prior clinical trial. Ann Thorac Surg. 2011;92:1406–13.
3. Kirklin JK, Naftel DC, Kormos RL, Stevenson LW, Pagani FD, Miller MA, Baldwin JT, Young JB. Fifth INTERMACS annual report: Risk factor analysis from more than 6,000 mechanical circulatory support patients. J Heart Lung Transplant. 2013;32:141–56.
4. Park SJ, Milano CA, Tatooles AJ, Rogers JG, Adamson RM, Steidley DE, Ewald GA, Sundareswaran KS, Farrar DJ, Slaughter MS. Outcomes in advanced heart failure patients with left ventricular assist devices for destination therapy. Circ Heart Fail. 2012;5:241–8.
5. Slaughter MS, Rogers JG, Milano CA, Russell SD, Conte JV, Feldman D, Sun B, Tatooles AJ, Delgado RM, Long JW, Wozniak TC, Ghumman W, Farrar DJ, Frazier OH. Advanced heart failure treated with continuous-flow left ventricular assist device. N Engl J Med. 2009;361:2241–51.
6. Bourque K, Dague C, Farrar D, Harms K, Tamez D, Cohn W, Tuzun E, Poirier V, Frazier OH. In vivo assessment of a rotary left ventricular assist device-induced artificial pulse in the proximal and distal aorta. Artif Organs. 2007;30(8):638–42.
7. Farrar DJ, Bourque K, Dague CP, Cotter CJ, Poirier VL. Design features, developmental status, and experimental results with the Heartmate III centrifugal left ventricular assist system with a magnetically levitated rotor. ASAIO J. 2007;53(3):310–5.
8. Dowling RD, Gray Jr LA, Etoch SW, Laks H, Marelli D, Samuels L, Entwistle J, Couper G, Vlahakes GJ, Frazier OH. Initial experience with the AbioCor implantable replacement heart system. J Thorac Cardiovasc Surg. 2004;127(1):131–41.
9. Pae WE, Connell JM, Adelowo A, Boehmer JP, Korfer R, El-Banayosy HR, Vigano M, Pavie A. Does total implantability reduce infection with the use of a left ventricular assist device? The lionheart experience in Europe. J Heart Lung Transplant. 2007;26:219–29.
10. Sundareswaran KS, Reichenbach SH, Masterson KB, Butler KC, Farrar DJ. Low bearing wear in explanted HeartMate II left ventricular assist devices after chronic clinical support. ASAIO J. 2013;59(1):41–5.
11. Karalis A, Joannopoulos JD, Soljacic M. Efficient wireless non-radiative mid-range energy transfer. Ann Phys. 2008;323:34–48.

Index

A
AbioCor fully implantable total artificial
heart device, 9
Ablations, 7, 18
Activities of daily living, 24, 32
Adamson technique, 19
Advanced age, 43
Advanced heart failure, 24
Adverse event(s), 43, 47, 52, 55–57
Adverse event rates, 41, 47
Age of increased risk, 41
Amplatzer occluder devices, 19
Anderson–Darling test, 47
Anticoagulation, 84
Antiplatelet agent, 81
Aortic aneurysm, 20
Aortic insufficiency, 12, 85
Aortic valve, 18, 19
    aortic valvular regurgitation, 19
    patch closure, 48
Arteriovenous malformations, 89
Artificial pulse, 134, 135
Atrial fibrillation, 20
Axial flow, 28, 31, 37

B
Baseline patient characteristics, 47–48
Best Practices Initiative, 12, 13
Biventricular, 137–139
    failure, 76
    pacing, 46
    pumping, 18
Bleeding, 7, 9–12
Blood pressure, 90–91

Bridge to transplant (BTT), 24–29, 31, 34
    indications, 114
Bulk flow, 20

C
Cardiac transplantation, 43, 98–108
Cardiogenic shock, 43, 45, 55, 75
Cardiopulmonary bypass, 83
Cardiovascular disease, 2
Centers for Medicare and Medicaid
Services, 44
Chronic inotropic infusion, 2
Collapsible impeller, 140
Comparison of patients, 54
Congestive heart failure, 43
Continuous flow devices, 18
Continuous flow pump, 9, 10, 16, 18, 20
Cost, 99, 106–108
Coumadin, 10
Current opportunities for
improvement, 5–8

D
Designing the perfect pump, 15–16
Destination therapy (DT), 5, 24–30, 33,
34, 41–57, 114
    risk score, 43
Dilated cardiomyopathy, 20
Driveline, 88
    infection, 33
DT. *See* Destination therapy (DT)
Durable pulsatile systems, 20
Duration of support, 48, 50

S. Kyo (ed.), *Ventricular Assist Devices in Advanced-Stage Heart Failure*,
DOI 10.1007/978-4-431-54466-1, © Springer Japan 2014

Made in the USA
Monee, IL
07 July 2026

56550841R00098